THE
LIFERAFT
SURVIVAL
GUIDE
HOW TO PREPARE
FOR THE WORST

EMERGENCY FLOWCHART

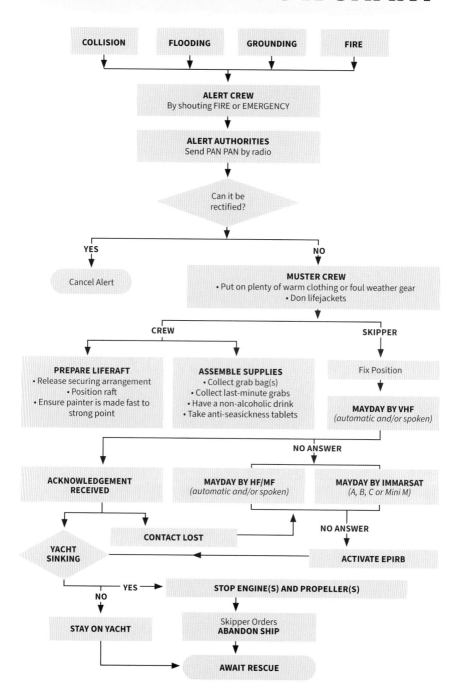

FRANCES &
MICHAEL HOWORTH

THE LIFERAFT SURVIVAL GUIDE

HOW TO PREPARE FOR THE WORST

ADLARD
COLES

LONDON · OXFORD · NEW YORK · NEW DELHI · SYDNEY

ADLARD COLES
Bloomsbury Publishing Plc
50 Bedford Square, London, WC1B 3DP, UK
29 Earlsfort Terrace, Dublin 2, Ireland

BLOOMSBURY, ADLARD COLES and the Adlard Coles logo are trademarks of
Bloomsbury Publishing Plc

First published as *The Grab Bag Book*, 2002
This revised edition published 2023

A catalogue record for this book is available from the British Library

Library of Congress Cataloguing-in-Publication data has been applied for

ISBN: PB: 978-1-3994-0150-0; ePub: 978-1-3994-0151-7; ePDF: 978-1-3994-0148-7

2 4 6 8 10 9 7 5 3 1

Typeset in Source Sans Pro by Nerine Dorman
Printed and bound in India by Replika Press Pvt Ltd

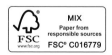

MIX
Paper from
responsible sources
FSC® C016779

To find out more about our authors and books visit www.bloomsbury.com and
sign up for our newsletter

Note: While all reasonable care has been taken in the publication of this book, the publisher takes no
responsibility for the use of the methods or products described in the book.

CONTENTS

AUTHORS' NOTE

THROUGHOUT THIS BOOK the word 'skipper' is used to describe the person in charge of the boat. The skipper is not necessarily the owner of the vessel, though they may be.

The use of the masculine and feminine pronoun is arbitrary. It does not indicate that any gender is preferred or desired for any job or function.

The term 'yacht' is used throughout the book, and this can be any pleasure vessel of any size, whether sail, motor or both. A registered pleasure vessel of 13.7m (45ft) or more in length is classified as a Class XII vessel in the UK by the Maritime and Coastguard Agency (MCA). Various regulations apply to Class XII ships, and these are highlighted in Chapter 2.

Yachts that cease to be 'pleasure vessels' and/or Class XII vessels are subject to different legal requirements and codes of practice. Those regulations are not considered in this book and must be reviewed before any safety equipment is purchased.

This book complies with the International Maritime Organization (IMO) resolution A.657(16).

Our thanks to:

Rob Priestley JRCC Commander HM Coastguard Operations
Peter Broadhurst, Inmarsat
Alistair Hackett, Ocean Safety
Mikele D'Arcangelo ACR
Sam Kelly, Head of Training at the Maritime Skills Academy
Dr Andrew Wolfle, MRCGP

1 BEING PREPARED

Common yachting folklore warns us all against thinking about a disaster at sea on the basis that if you do, it is sure to happen. But as the skipper of a yacht, you must be prepared for every eventuality, and it is your duty to make sure all your crew are, too.

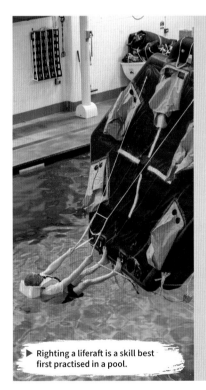

▶ Righting a liferaft is a skill best first practised in a pool.

This book is all about:

- Surviving the disaster of abandoning ship.
- Being mentally and physically prepared for the sailor's ultimate nightmare.
- Why you need to supplement the equipment found inside your liferaft.
- Selecting equipment for your grab bag.

It is NOT about:

- The brand of liferaft or EPIRB you should buy.
- Dealing with the accident or emergency that caused the disaster.

It is written for:

- Skipper and crew aboard any private vessel.
- Any size or type of boat.
- Any voyage from across the bay to around the world.

▶ *Proper Preparation*

AS A RESPONSIBLE skipper, part of the planning for a passage includes ensuring the correct safety equipment is carried aboard your yacht. It is not easy to part with hard earned money for an item of equipment that you doubt will be used, and may even be thrown away after a few years still unopened. It is all too easy to cut corners at the purchasing stage and buy only the barest minimum. Sadly, when the unimaginable catastrophe happens it will probably be too late to go back and purchase that safety item you previously rejected as an unnecessary expense. As author Lee Child once said, 'Hope for the best, but plan for the worst'.

The danger is greater the further you go offshore, because of the higher risk of being at sea in rough weather, but at least you probably cannot run aground in the middle of an ocean. A shipwreck, however, can happen anywhere, at any time. If you do have to take to your liferaft, what can you do to improve your chances of being rescued, without injury or loss of life? Read this book at your passage planning stage to decide what to select for your emergency bag – and store this book in your grab bag so you will have it with you in the liferaft.

▶ *Training*

The importance of training cannot be emphasised enough. A practical sea survival course to give at least the skipper, and ideally all the crew, real-world experience with a liferaft, and this book for reference is an ideal combination.

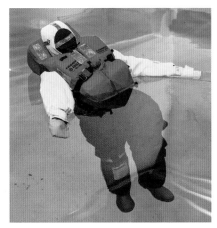

▶ Immersion suit.

Confidence comes from training and knowledge.

A typical Royal Yachting Association (RYA) Basic Sea Survival Course for example will cover:

- Liferafts and the equipment they contain.
- Launching a liferaft.
- Survival techniques.
- Medical aspects of sea survival.
- Search and rescue techniques.
- And most important of all – a two hour practical session in the water with a liferaft.

Practical liferaft experience is also part of the Standards of Training, Certification and Watchkeeping (STCW) Basic Safety Training course, required by anyone looking to work on commercial vessels over 24m (78.7ft), including superyachts.

While a practical course is excellent, there is not time in a single day to cover all the information to help you decide what to pack in a grab bag and how to survive an abandon ship. That is where this

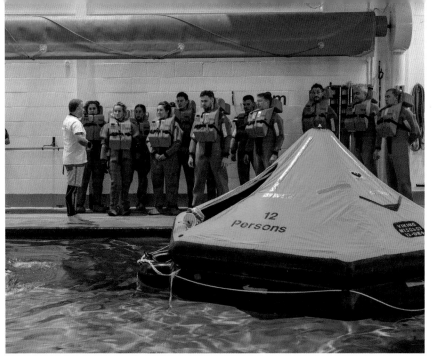

▶ Certified training is absolutely vital for anyone looking to work on commercial vessels.

book will help. It should be read by every crewmember, re-read regularly, and used for training exercises.

Research has shown that when disaster strikes 75 per cent of people will be stunned and bewildered. Those who have been trained to expect and to cope with such situations will fall back on well-learned patterns of behaviour. A trained crew will work together to leave the yacht safely, carrying with them the maximum equipment to aid their survival.

It is vital that the skipper demonstrates strong leadership and appropriate action both before and after abandonment. It would be nice to think that once you are safely aboard your liferaft your worst troubles are over and you will be rescued almost immediately. With modern communications, help should be on its way, but you still have to survive until it arrives. What is already packed inside your liferaft and what you additionally take with you are your keys to survival.

▶ Liferaft Emergency Packs

Horror stories about the survival gear found in liferafts abound. It's not just a question of the lack of equipment, or the missing items, but also the quality of the supplies. Even in the best of liferafts the supplies included are limited. It all comes

 Remember: *No one is a survivor until they have been rescued or have reached safety by their own efforts.*

down to money and weight; the more supplies that are packed with a liferaft, the heavier it is, the larger the outer container needed and the more expensive it becomes. Most rafts for the leisure market are sold with a choice of packs, with the most basic and cheapest being a selection of simple items to maintain the raft – and not necessarily of high quality. Pray you never have to survive for long with just a basic pack.

▶ Why You Need a Grab Bag

Even in the best situation for abandoning ship, when you have a little time, these precious minutes are far more likely to be spent trying to save your yacht rather than choosing what to take with you.

You are unlikely to be in the best frame of mind to make sensible decisions, nor will you necessarily have the equipment that will aid you best in a liferaft. You need to have thought about your choices ahead of time, gone shopping online or physically, and been alongside to take delivery of your order.

Your grab bag should contain everything essential to your survival in a liferaft. If you do not have a liferaft and propose to use your dinghy in an emergency, it is even more important to have some form of abandon ship bag, as your dinghy is unlikely to have even the most basic of emergency supplies.

▶ Your Yacht and its Equipment

No two situations are ever the same, but if a yacht is sinking there is one overriding priority: the saving of life. It is too late at this point to discover that the liferaft is out of date for a service, the EPIRB is registered in the name of another yacht and the spare flares were landed last weekend.

Good seamanship, knowledge and common sense will help ensure safety

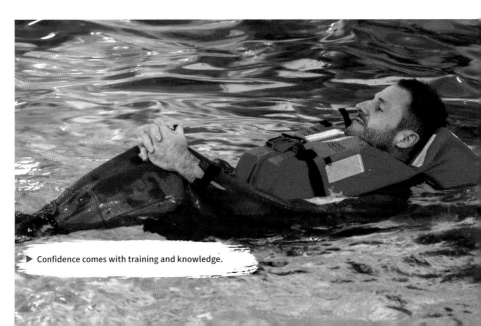

▶ Confidence comes with training and knowledge.

at sea. With planning and forethought, many a disaster can be prevented but sadly not all. The training needed by you and your crew together with the equipment you choose for your yacht depends, to a large extent, on the areas in which you sail or plan to sail, the weather conditions you are likely to encounter and, to a lesser extent, upon the size of your yacht. A large yacht may need more of, or a larger size of, some equipment than her smaller sister, but most of the items will be identical, if they are sailing in the same areas.

▶ Global Maritime Distress and Safety Systems (GMDSS)

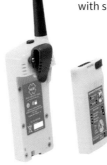

▶ Waterproof handheld survival VHF radio with removable battery.

Since 1999, when the Global Maritime Distress and Safety System (GMDSS) became worldwide, going to sea has been much safer. It is now much more likely that a yacht in distress will receive assistance and that time spent by crew in a liferaft will be much shorter. It is much more likely to be hours, rather than days, before rescue. No longer does a lack of contact before abandoning ship mean your chance of rescue in a remote area is minimal.

GMDSS is a ship-to-shore communications system, where a vessel in distress can alert a land-based Rescue Co-ordination Centre (RCC), which then co-ordinates the rescue. It is both proactive, ie sending out navigational and meteorological information, and reactive, ie being able to send a distress, urgency or safety message. It is an international system using terrestrial and satellite technology together with ship-board radio systems, ensuring that vessels (wherever they are in the world) can communicate with shore stations and other ships.

The equipment does not require specialist radio operators and an important part of the system is the automatic way in which it transmits and receives distress alerts, either using conventional radio or the Inmarsat satellite system. GMDSS is not just for emergency and distress messages; it is also used for urgency broadcasts, medical assistance, reporting back safety information and routine ship-to-ship and ship-to-shore communications.

GMDSS is not just a more expensive radio that calls and listens on designated frequencies and saves the authorities from listening out on special distress frequencies; it is a complete system with several elements including satellite communication, weather and navigation information and secondary distress signalling devices.

Generally, all GMDSS-compliant vessels carry a 406 MHz Emergency Position Indicating Radio Beacon (EPIRB), a VHF radio capable of transmitting and receiving Digital Selective Calling (DSC) and radiotelephony, a navigational telex (NAVTEX) receiver for weather and transport information, a Search and Rescue Transponder (SART), and two-way VHF portable radios.

At present, it is not compulsory for a small private yacht to carry GMDSS equipment, but all boats should include some if not all the elements of the system. The decision on which of the elements to fit will depend upon the nature of that yacht's voyaging but, at the very least, every yacht should carry a VHF with DSC. Where a yacht is planning an ocean passage, MF/HF DSC equipment should be considered, as VHF range is limited.

GMDSS is fully implemented on commercial vessels over 300gt and an increasing number of other vessels. These vessels are no longer obliged to listen out on channel 16 or 2182 kHz. Coastal stations will continue to listen on the designated emergency channels but, in a busy traffic area, a poor signal may be lost in the background noise. It is highly recommended that all boats have GMDSS-compliant equipment with a DSC controller to attract attention when making a Mayday call. GMDSS is essential for any offshore yacht.

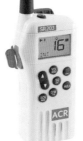

► Waterproof handheld survival VHF radio.

ability to include other information such as:

- The yacht's identification number.
- The reason for the call.
- The yacht's position.
- The channel you want to speak on.

For routine calls a VHF DSC radio operates in a very similar way to a telephone, in that you can call another yacht or coastal station directly without involving anyone else. Each DSC radio is assigned a unique nine digit number or Maritime Mobile Service Identity (MMSI), similar to a telephone number. It is no longer necessary to try to contact another yacht by calling on channel 16, which would clutter up the channel and may not get through if the crew of the other yacht are not listening.

Where DSC really excels is in the simplicity of making a call in an emergency. Depending upon the equipment fitted, a distress call can be initiated by pressing one or two pre-programmed Distress Alert buttons, some-thing that all crew can be taught in seconds. The alert will be heard immediately by all DSC-equipped vessels and shore stations in range and the information they receive will include the yacht's identity and position (most DSC modems are interconnected to the yacht's GPS receiver), as well as the time.

Benefits of DSC

DSC is a tone signalling system, which operates on VHF channel 70 with the

VHF vs Mobile Cellular Phone

It is easy to understand why a mobile phone is not going to be useful in calling

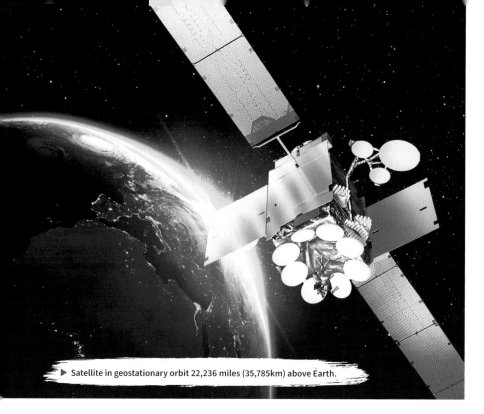

▶ Satellite in geostationary orbit 22,236 miles (35,785km) above Earth.

for help in the middle of the Atlantic, but there a several practical reasons why it is not a replacement for a VHF, even where there is mobile coverage:

- The Coastguard may not be able to re-establish contact if connection is lost.
- Cell towers cover areas of land, not sea, so coverage is unreliable offshore – sometimes you may get a signal miles 25 miles (40km) offshore and other times only 10 miles (16km) offshore.
- Mobile phones communicate directly with one person rather than broadcasting generally, so other vessels will not be aware of an emergency.
- The freely available app What3Words gives a precise location for every 3m

square of the world's seas and oceans, however, a yacht does not remain still. Your DSC will continually update its location, but constantly updating a location manually while dealing with an emergency is not a good combination, and will quickly drain a battery.

Despite the obvious problems with using a mobile phone for a distress alert, it can be used in an emergency. Make sure the What3Words app is downloaded on every mobile phone aboard the yacht, it is an excellent additional tool.

Satellite communications

Reliable, always-on satellite connectivity with flexible airtime plans is now within the reach of many yachts. The latest

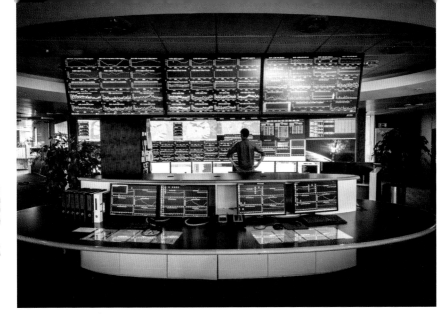

▶ Inmarsat – Network Operations Centre (NOC).

external antennas are compact and lightweight and combine with a below deck terminal, hard-wired handset and Wi-Fi router to give crew aboard Wi-Fi access to the internet and the ability to make and receive calls. Inmarsat's global service is delivered using the Inmarsat I-4 satellites over the reliable L-band satellite network, maintaining over 99.9 per cent availability. The reassurance of voice and data connection for emergencies, business, support services, passage planning, weather updates and staying in touch with family and friends back home can improve life on board and enhance safety.

In an emergency a satellite phone has the same problem as a cellular phone, in that there is only communication with one person rather than broadcasting generally to all nearby vessels. But a mobile

▶ Most EPIRBs have a 10-year battery life.

satellite phone is a valuable addition for contacting help for two reasons:

- It does not stop working offshore.
- If radio contact is impossible then the reassurance of speaking to someone off the yacht is invaluable.

▶ Emergency Position Indicating Radio Beacon (EPIRB)

An Emergency Position Indicating Radio Beacon (EPIRB) is a small, portable, battery-powered transmitter that can automatically send an emergency signal and locating signal to rescue services. They have been in use since the 1980s and all vessels required to carry

GMDSS, regardless of the sea area they sail in, must carry EPIRBs. It is probably the most important piece of equipment to pack in your grab bag.

EPIRBs take advantage of communications satellites to give complete global coverage and transmit a coded message via the free-to-use, multinational COSPAS-SARSAT network. COSPAS-SARSAT is an international satellite-based search and rescue system established by the US, Russia, Canada and France to locate emergency radio beacons transmitting on emergency frequencies. The signal frequency (406 MHz) has been designated internationally for use only for distress. The 406 MHz EPIRB is designed to operate via satellite and Earth stations to the nearest rescue co-ordination centre.

Older EPIRBs operating on the 121.5/243 MHz frequency are no longer monitored by the International Cospas-Sarsat System. Alerts from these devices using 121.5/243 MHz EPIRBs will no longer be acted upon by SAR authorities unless independently confirmed by two independent non-satellite sources.

But EPIRBs still transmit a low powered homing signal via 121.5 MHz and these help SAR vessels and any aircraft to home in on the beacon's location. Civil aircraft, especially those on oceanic routes, still monitor the 121.5 MHz frequency and much useful corroborative information is reported by over-flying aircraft.

New medium earth orbiting satellites using the European Galileo system have cut the time a distress message takes to reach those monitoring them. There is now no need for second satellite pass verification. This means an alert sounds at an MRCC within five minutes of the EPIRB being activated.

The only downside of an EPIRB was not knowing if the authorities had received the signal, but units

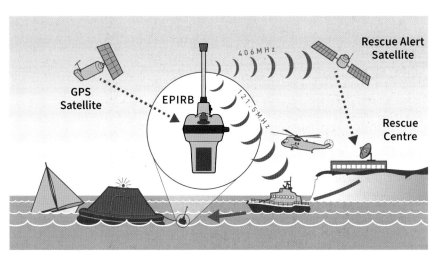

▶ Emergency Position Indicating Radio Beacons (EPIRB) send emergency and locating signals to rescue services.

manufactured after 2022 can receive a message that their alert has been received.

Automatic Identification System (AIS) EPIRB

An EPIRB installed on or after 1 July 2022 must have an internal Automatic Identification System (AIS) frequency, along with the 406 MHz channel and a GNSS (GPS) receiver fitted. The AIS channel transmits an SOS signal that will be received directly by all nearby vessels equipped with AIS within about 4 miles (6.4km). The GNSS technology adds location data, enabling the nearest vessel (or vessels) to come and help immediately.

Since EPIRBs were first introduced more than 52,000 people have been rescued following an EPIRB alert. On average seven lives are saved every day.

One sailor who owes his life to an EPIRB is Pablo Pirenack. He left the USA to fulfil a lifelong ambition to sail a small yacht single-handed across the Atlantic. He got more than he bargained for when a hurricane battered his 8m (26ft) yacht to bits and he took to his liferaft. It was his EPIRB that saved him by enabling a gas tanker to come to his rescue, just 26 hours after he first hit the transmit button. His story is a salutary lesson to one and all who cross the seas in small craft.

Other sailors have not been so lucky. Jennifer Appel and Tasha Fuiava drifted powerless for months while trying to sail *Sea Nymph*, a 15m (49ft) sailboat, 2,700 miles (4,300km) from Hawaii to Tahiti. The pair had an EPIRB, but never turned it on. Appel believed the beacons should be used only when sailors are

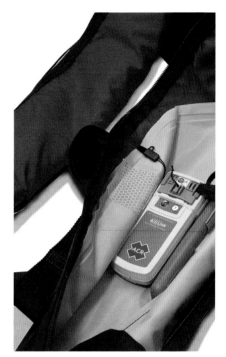

▶ Personal man overboard beacon.

in imminent danger or at risk of death within 24 hours. She said, 'EPIRB calls are for people who are in an immediate life-threatening scenario.' She felt that it would be shameful to call on the United States Coast Guard (USCG) resources when not in imminent peril as someone else could perish because of it. The retired Coastguard officer, who was responsible for search and rescue operations, said that there is no shame in using an EPIRB in any true emergency and in this case stated, 'The women would have been found very quickly if only they had turned on the beacon'. He added, 'Had they turned it on, a signal should have been received very, very quickly and we would have known a whole lot sooner that this vessel was in distress'.

▶ PLBs

Personal Locator Beacons (PLBs) are personal electronic transmitters used to alert rescuers that there has been a life-threatening situation with a need for someone to be rescued. When activated, they work in the same way as EPIRBs, by sending out a signal on either a 406 MHz frequency or the Local Area System using 121.5 MHz, VHF DSC and/or AIS if included.

However, there are several differences between PLBs and EPIRBs:

- PLBs are small so they can be easily carried/worn, but unlike EPIRBs they may not float.
- PLBs transmit for a minimum of 24 hours and can be stored for six years, while EPIRBs transmit for at least 48 hours and can typically be stored for 10 years.
- An EPIRB is registered to a vessel, whereas a PLB is registered to a person.
- PLBs cannot be designed to be automatically activated – they are too easy to drop or mishandle.
- PLBs are an excellent personal Man Over Board (MOB) device, assuming the victim is wearing one. This is a job that an EPIRB cannot do

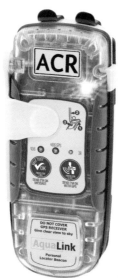

▶ **Personal man overboard beacon.**

unless it can be thrown to the person in the water.

Distress signals generated by GMDSS equipment are received by rescue co-ordination centres and are always acted upon. AIS SARTs and PLBs are not part of GMDSS. This means that when they are activated, the authorities know nothing about the associated vessel and the alert is not treated as a distress signal. Because of their prevalence, they will be investigated in UK waters, but signals may not be followed-up elsewhere in the world.

▶ Lessons Learned from Disasters

Two yacht races have had a major impact on safety: the 1979 Fastnet Race and the 1998 Sydney—Hobart Yacht Race. The Fastnet disaster, which cost the lives of 15 sailors, caused a major upheaval in yacht design in the 1980s. The Sydney—Hobart tragedy cost six lives and the findings of John Abernethy, the Australian Coroner, are still having repercussions. The recommendations of that coroner, though intended for racing boats, should be considered by any cruising yacht when selecting safety equipment and are as relevant today as in the late 1990s. They included the requirement that all:

- Crew wear a personal EPIRB when on deck, in all weather conditions.
- Crew are trained in the use of personal EPIRBs.
- Yachts carry on board a 406 MHz EPIRB.
- Yachts' batteries be of the closed or gel cell type.
- Crew who are on deck during rough weather should wear clothing that will protect them from hypothermia.
- Crew use personal flotation devices (PFDs) other than the 'Mae West' type lifejackets.
- Crew have with them a personal strobe light when on deck in all weather conditions.

The Coroner gave further recommendations concerning liferafts and training, which are included in the next chapter.

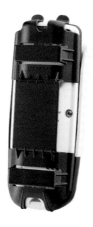

▶ **Personal man overboard beacon and bracket.**

It all went wrong

While attempting to sail across the Atlantic, *Cheeki Rafiki*, a 12m (40ft) Bénéteau sailing yacht, lost her keel about 720 nautical miles southeast of Nova Scotia and subsequently capsized in a Force 7 storm. Her EPIRB was never activated, but rescue services were able to locate her upturned hull before it sank because two PLB devices had sent emergency signals. Sadly, the crew of four were never found. US Navy divers boarded the still-floating wreck and confirmed her liferaft was still secured to its storage location. Clearly the crew had not brought it out on deck. We will never know why the EPIRB was not activated, or the liferaft deployed, but perhaps it would be good to use the story as a crew training exercise to consider what should be done on your yacht in a similar emergency.

Do not switch your EPIRB off

In late 2022, the UK's HM Coastguard and three merchant vessels were involved in the rescue of a lone sailor from the Atlantic Ocean, after the yacht lost its mast in stormy conditions.

The Coastguard's Joint Rescue Co-ordination Centre (JRCC) received two distress beacon alerts from the yacht 700 nautical miles west of Ireland. These signals from the EPIRBs were the only means the sailor had of communicating that he was in distress. All other communication methods had been destroyed during the event that led to the dismasting of the yacht. The American-flagged vessel had extensive damage and was drifting in very poor weather conditions.

A request was made to deploy aircraft from both RAF Brize Norton and RAF Lossiemouth. There are nine submarine-hunting P-8 Poseidons at RAF Lossiemouth, tasked with keeping a watchful eye on the North Atlantic, and the RAF wasted no time in scrambling to assist. Wing Commander Ben Livesey, OC CXX Squadron, P-8 Poseidon, said: 'The power of the weather once again highlighted the importance of a meaningful search and rescue capability. Co-operative events such as these demonstrate the way crews from across the RAF can work together to deliver great effect'.

Together with the crew aboard an Atlas A400M from RAF Brize Norton, the Poseidon P-8 team helped locate the yacht 700 nautical miles west of Ireland. Having identified the stricken yacht, using co-ordinates provided by the JRCC, they dropped liferafts into the water nearby.

At the same time, HM Coastguard was broadcasting to all shipping within 300 miles (483km) and three vessels responded, altering their courses to intercept the yacht.

Rescue from that point on should have been simple, despite poor sea conditions. Unfortunately, the yachtsman switched off his EPIRB beacon as soon as he saw the aircraft make a low pass over his position. Without a radio, a SART or an EPIRB broadcasting the location, the yacht was effectively lost again.

Surface conditions on scene were rough and it was some 48 hours later when the yachtsman was finally relocated. After four unsuccessful rescue attempts by merchant ships, the crew of the Aframax tanker *Amax Anthem* tried again and finally succeeded in getting the survivor safely aboard their ship.

Afterwards Rob Priestley, JRCC Commander, said: 'This became a lengthy and complex search and rescue mission because the yacht had no other communications method and with his EPIRB turned off, that made finding him again with a ship, rather difficult'.

▶ Shoreside Preparation

Even with the most comprehensive communications equipment, a distress call may be unsuccessful in attracting attention or providing enough information for the rescue services. It is vital that someone ashore knows where you are sailing and what survival equipment you carry. Before any passage, fill in a Voyage Details Plan (see Appendix 1 on page 125) and give it to your nominated shoreside contact. It will give them all the details they need to help set into motion a Search and Rescue, in the event of your yacht failing to arrive at her destination at the expected time.

In July 2020, the UK Voluntary Safety Information Scheme (CG66), which recorded data about vessels, owners and shore contacts was scrapped and RYA SafeTrx is now recommended in its place. SafeTrx is freely available and provides a similar, more enhanced, Search and Rescue (SAR) database managed by the RYA but open to all boat users, not just RYA members. It is important to note that due to data protection rules the CG66 database was not transferred to SafeTRx.

RYA SafeTrx allows you to register your vessel, its communications and safety equipment and your emergency contacts using an app or on the RYA's website. The app is freely available for iPhones running iOS 8.0 or later, and on Android phones with Android OS 4.2 or later. Using the app, you can also plan and track your trip on your smartphone using Wi-Fi or a mobile connection and the device's GPS to determine location. In the event of the app failing to report your safe arrival by the logged ETA, the system will send an escalating series of alerts culminating in an SMS to your designated emergency contact, who can then contact the Coastguard to initiate a SAR. Those without a smartphone can enter data via the website at safetrx.rya.org.uk, but tracking and reporting functions are not available.

While RYA SafeTrx is a valuable tool, it does have limitations. Primarily, it is designed for those sailing locally on single voyages not cruising. Cruisers should continue to report their voyages to UK Coastguard via VHF. Additionally, use of the tracking and reporting functions are battery heavy and rely on an internet connection, both of which can be a problem.

When an emergency occurs, the importance of accurate up-to-date information cannot be emphasised

enough. The action the rescue services take will be influenced by many things, including the size, shape and number of persons aboard the vessel requiring help. As well as having a nominated shoreside contact who can initiate an emergency call and supply all the details about the yacht, it is important to fill in all the official paperwork.

When the authorities get an emergency alert, one of the things they do is check for details of the yacht. Chasing emergency contacts after a yacht (and the EPIRB with it) has been sold on to new owners is a major headache and will delay correct response to an emergency. In the UK, If a yacht is not recorded in the Ship Register, the Coastguard encourages owners of private yachts that are less than 24m (78.7ft) to use the Small Ships Register to record their yacht.

As Sam Kelly, Head of Training at the Maritime Skills Academy, says 'Failing to prepare is preparing to fail'.

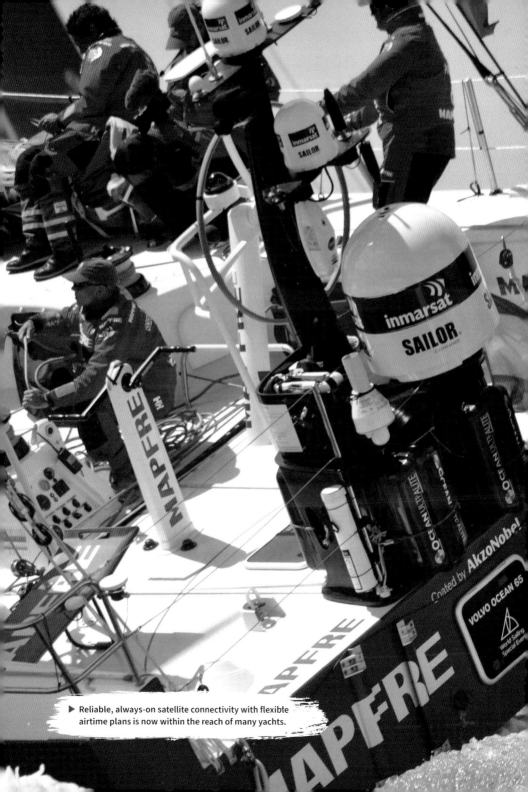

▶ Reliable, always-on satellite connectivity with flexible airtime plans is now within the reach of many yachts.

2 YOUR LIFERAFT AND ITS CONTENTS

A liferaft is designed as a last resort to keep the crew of a boat alive after their vessel has sunk until help arrives. It should provide environmental protection, even in rough seas, and aid location by creating a larger target for the rescuers to find. It can never be as comfortable as your yacht, but it should be a lot better than floating in the water supported by a lifejacket. A liferaft should never be used unless it is certain that the boat herself cannot be saved. It is not a better refuge than a yacht, nor can it be considered safer in rough seas than the much larger parent vessel. Remember the old adage: **Never step down into a liferaft.**

▶ Choosing a Liferaft

LIFERAFT MANUFACTURERS DO not make things easy. While one liferaft may be more expensive than another, this may be due to the survival pack contents rather than the construction of the raft itself. It is extremely unlikely that you will get the chance to test a range of liferafts, and unless you go to a boat show you will probably be buying blind, trusting a salesman or a manufacturer's reputation. Worst of all, you will, in all likelihood, be parting with your money to buy something you will never see open until the first service.

Various organisations have laid down standards of manufacture, design and equipment to be carried in liferafts. The International Maritime Organization (IMO) have, in their Safety Of Life At Sea Convention (SOLAS), created the highest standard. World Sailing Special Regulations have produced the next highest standard required by pleasure craft engaged in racing. Liferafts for leisure sailors are governed by the International Organization for Standardization (ISO) under ISO 9650, introduced in 2005 to ensure minimum standards of liferaft survival kit and performance aboard non-commercial yachts under 24m (78.7ft).

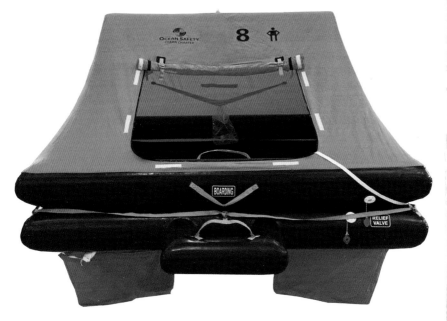

▶ The Ocean Charter ISO liferaft.

It is still possible to buy a non-approved liferaft that may be similar to an ISO-compliant liferaft, but with more basic fixtures and fittings, minimal equipment and no guarantee of the standard of build. For American boaters the officiating body is the United States Coastguard (USCG).

Buying any liferaft is all about choices. Sea conditions can be as rough close to shore as in the middle of the ocean. The main difference when going further afield is not the quality or style of your liferaft but the need to carry more survival gear.

- Should you choose, a SOLAS, ISO 9650 or USCG specified model?
- Would the cheapest model be sufficient?
- What size do you select?
- Should it be stored in a container or a valise?
- Which survival pack do you buy?
- What about renting instead of buying?

▶ *Liferaft Types*

Apart from a SOLAS liferaft (page 18), there are four main types of survival craft used aboard private yachts:

Inflatable dinghy

- Can be pressed into service in an emergency.
- Only of use if stored inflated on deck.
- Always second best.
- Only really useful in very calm conditions.
- Easily capsizes and floats inverted in heavy seas.

Dual-purpose tender/liferaft

- Special tender manufactured to convert to liferaft use, such as the USA manufactured Portland Pudgy.

17

- Liferaft conversion with an optional inflatable exposure canopy and other survival gear.
- As expensive as some stand-alone liferaft.
- To change from one function to another is time consuming.
- It can be rowed, motored or sailed towards shipping lanes or shore.

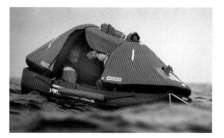

▶ Portland Pudgy lifeboat on test in the North Sea.

Coastal liferaft: ISO 9650 Type 2

- For sailing areas with moderate conditions such as coastal waters, estuaries, rivers and lakes.
- For temperatures of 0–65°C (32–149°F) with single floor.
- Twin independent buoyancy tubes.
- Manual canopy.
- Standard survival kit.

Offshore liferaft: ISO 9650 Type 1

- For long voyages or cruises and rough conditions (excluding extreme conditions such as hurricanes).
- Twin independent buoyancy tubes.
- Group A: designed for temperatures of 0–65°C (32–149°F) with single floor.

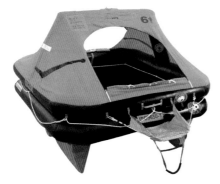

▶ Charter ISO inflated liferaft front.

- Group B: designed for temperatures of -15–65°C (5–149°F) with insulating double floor.
- Automatic canopy.
- Two variations of survival kit depending on expected time until rescue.

▶ SOLAS Liferaft

Bulkier, heavier and of course more expensive than a liferaft designed specifically for private vessels, a commercial standard SOLAS-compliant model is highly recommended for yachts planning to go more than 150 miles (241km) from the coast. It is required for vessels racing that far offshore under World Sailing Special Regulations.

A statement made by the Coroner following the disastrous 1998 Sydney–Hobart Race should be considered when choosing a raft:

'The recommendation of a liferaft complying with the SOLAS requirements is not, as one submission states, for "A possible slight gain in people comfort in the unusual circumstance of a crew having to take to the raft". It is so that, if the unusual circumstance does arise, the crew will have the best opportunity of survival, and they are entitled to that.'

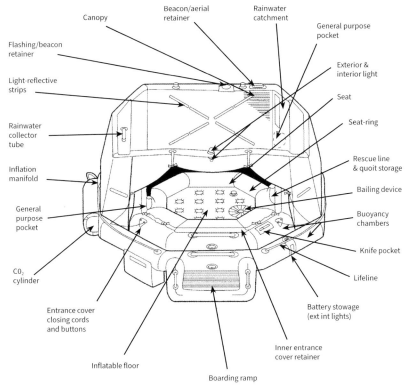

Canopy
Beacon/aerial retainer
Rainwater catchment
General purpose pocket
Flashing/beacon retainer
Exterior & interior light
Light-reflective strips
Seat
Rainwater collector tube
Seat-ring
Inflation manifold
Rescue line & quoit storage
General purpose pocket
Bailing device
Buoyancy chambers
CO_2 cylinder
Knife pocket
Lifeline
Entrance cover closing cords and buttons
Battery stowage (ext int lights)
Inflatable floor
Inner entrance cover retainer
Boarding ramp

▶ Parts of a liferaft.

▶ *Size and Position*

Yacht liferafts are supplied in various sizes, depending upon the maximum number of crew intending to use it. A liferaft's buoyancy is directly related to the weight of the occupants and the ballast. Too much or too little and there is a risk of capsizing. With SOLAS or ISO 9650, where ballast is more than adequate, there is a good case for buying a raft that is intended for double the number of your expected crew, to give more room.

If a liferaft is to be of use in an emergency it must be immediately available, ideally stowed on deck or in a locker that opens from the deck.

- Assume that the raft will be needed rapidly and in heavy weather.
- Consider that the weakest person aboard may be deploying the raft.
- For on-deck storage, ensure the cradle is strong enough to hold the raft in rough weather.
- If stowed on the coach roof, plan how to move it to the deck edge in unstable conditions.
- If stowed on the pushpit, ensure the strapping arrangements are strong enough to hold the raft if it were submerged.
- Where stowed in a dedicated locker, consider access if the

yacht is at an unusual angle or moving violently.

- Valise-packed liferaft can expand or change shape over the course of a season, check it can be easily removed periodically.
- If fitted with a hydrostatic release, ensure the area around the liferaft is clear of obstruction so it can float free and the painter is correctly attached.

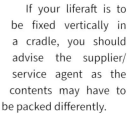

▶ A hydrostatic release unit.

Linked to the decision on location is choice of container:

A rigid plastic container

- For any liferaft kept on deck to protect from weather and knocks.
- Can be too heavy for a small person to move.

A fabric valise

- Lighter, less bulky and slightly cheaper.
- Only if protected from the elements in a deck locker or down below.

If your liferaft is to be fixed vertically in a cradle, you should advise the supplier/ service agent as the contents may have to be packed differently.

Many manufacturers now vacuum-bag their liferafts. This protects the raft from water ingress, reduces the size and lengthens the time before the first service is required.

Wherever you eventually choose to stow the liferaft, ensure everyone aboard is briefed on its location, the abandonment plan and how to deploy the

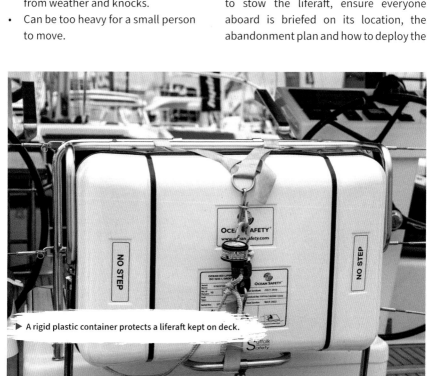

▶ A rigid plastic container protects a liferaft kept on deck.

raft. Make sure it has inflation instructions clearly written on it, or on an attached waterproof sticker, with the print large enough to be read without glasses. Check that these instructions are clear enough so even a complete novice would be able to understand them and launch the liferaft correctly.

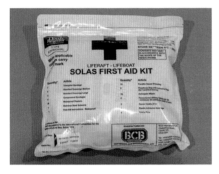

▶ Standardised emergency packs are usually stored inside a waterproof bag.

▶ Liferaft Emergency Packs

In general, the cheaper the liferaft the less equipment that is included. There are four standardised emergency packs available in order of comprehensiveness:

- ISO <24 hours
- ISO >24 hours
- SOLAS 'B'
- SOLAS 'A'

   Manufacturers typically offer a choice of packs and will include virtually any-thing else you want, for a price of course. The most basic emergency equipment only includes items to repair the raft, but even the most comprehensive SOLAS 'A'

pack will need to be augmented with a grab bag.

   Liferaft packs are usually stored inside a waterproof bag, attached within the raft, to prevent anything coming loose upon launching and inflation. The knife for cutting the painter is stowed separately, as are such items as a drogue and a rescue quoit.

▶ Liferaft Regulations for UK Registered Yachts

The Maritime and Coastguard Agency (MCA) is the regulatory body for UK registered vessels, including yachts. According to the MCA, a registered pleasure vessel of 13.7m (45ft) or more in length is classified as a Class XII ship in the UK. In 2020, Merchant Shipping Notice (MSN) 1676 (M) and various exemptions in Marine Guidance Note (MGN) 599 (M) covered liferafts.

- Yachts sailing less than 3 miles (4.8km) from the coast need not carry a liferaft.
- Yachts sailing over 3 miles (4.8km) from the coast must carry at least:
  - CE marked Category C rigid or inflatable dinghy ready to use.
  - Liferaft to ISO 9650 Type 2 if operating in air temperatures over 0°C (32°F).
- Yachts sailing over 20 miles (32.2km) from the coast must carry either:
  - ISO 9650 Type 1 Group B if operating in air temperatures over 0°C (32°F);
  - or ISO 9650 Type 2 Group A;
  - or SOLAS standards or Marine Equipment Directive (MED) approved.

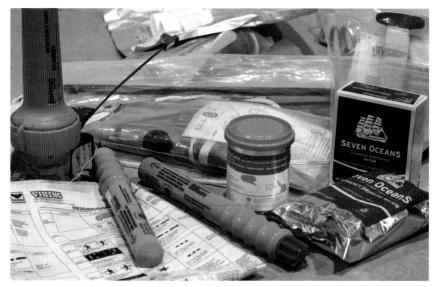

▶ All liferafts must be equipped with a suitable pack depending on how far off the coast a yacht is voyaging.

- Yachts over 24m (78.7ft) must have enough liferafts so, if one is lost or unusable, there is room for everyone aboard on the remaining liferafts unless:
  - Sailing less than 3 miles (4.8km) off the coast.
  - Closer than 60 miles (96.5km) from a safe haven.
  - In less than Beaufort force 4.

  Every liferaft must be:

- In approved fibre-reinforced plastic (FRP) containers stowed on the weather deck or in an open space, and fitted with float free arrangements so that the liferafts float free and inflate automatically.
- Yachts over 13.7m (45ft) but less than 24m (78.7ft) in length – in approved FRP containers or valise, stowed in a readily accessible and dedicated weather-tight locker, opening directly to the weather deck.

Distance Offshore	Minimum pack
3–20 miles (4.8–32km)	ISO (<24 hour)
20–150 miles (32–241km)	ISO (>24 hour) or SOLAS 'B' pack
150 miles (241km) or more	SOLAS 'A' pack *(If yacht is less than 24m (78.7ft), any pack plus grab bag to make up to SOLAS 'A' pack)*

Standard Liferaft Packs

UP TO 12 PERSONS	ISO <24 HOURS	ISO >24 HOURS	SOLAS 'B'	SOLAS 'A'
Rescue line and quoit	1	1	1	1
Safety knife	1	1	1	1
Bailer, buoyant	1	1	1	1
Sponge	2	2	2	2
Sea anchor	1	2	2	2
Paddle, buoyant	2	2	2	2
Can opener	–	–	–	3
Scissors, safety	–	–	–	1
First aid kit	–	ISO 9650	Category C	Category C
Whistle	–	1	–	1
Red parachute flare	2	4	2	4
Red handheld flares	3	6	3	6
Buoyant smoke signal	–	–	1	2
Flashlight, waterproof with spare batteries & bulb	2	2	1	1
Radar reflector or SART	–	–	1	1
Signalling mirror with instructions	1	1	1	1
DOT Rescue Signal Table	1	1	1	1
Fishing tackle	–	–	–	1
Food ration*	–	10,000kj pp	–	10,000kj pp
Drinking water*♦	–	1.5l pp	–	1.5l pp
Graduated drinking cup	–	–	–	1
Anti-seasickness tablets*	6pp	6pp	6pp	6pp
Seasickness bag*	1pp	1pp	1pp	1pp
Thermal protective aids	–	2	2	2
Survival instructions	1	1	1	1
Immediate action instructions	1	1	1	1
Pump or bellows	1	1	1	1
Repair kit	1	1	1	1

*: pp = amount required for each person the liferaft is permitted to carry
♦: Less water is required if the liferaft has desalting apparatus or a manual reverse osmosis desalinator

All liferafts must be equipped with a suitable pack depending upon how far off the coast the yacht is voyaging.

The minimum requirements for UK registered yachts are very sensible and should be given serious consideration when buying or renting a liferaft.

▶ Additions to Your Liferaft

It is worth considering storing some of your extra items inside the liferaft, especially if the supplied emergency pack included is very sparse. Prescription

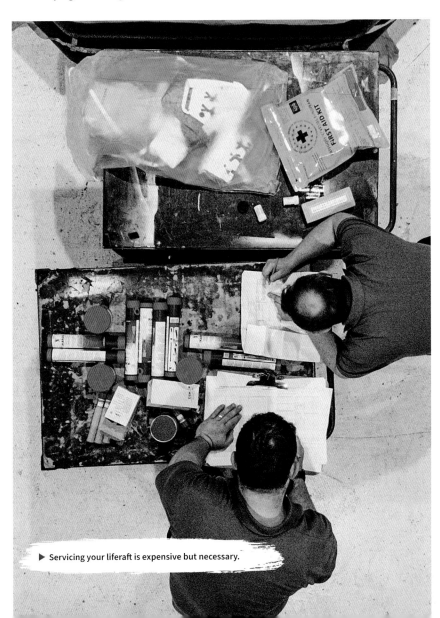

▶ Servicing your liferaft is expensive but necessary.

glasses, vital medication etc, can be added to a liferaft pack. This decision is best made when you purchase a new raft, as it may require a larger container to hold everything, but it can also be done at service time. The advantage is obviously that you know the gear will be with your liferaft. The downside is cost and that it will also make the raft heavier, so you need to be sure that the lightest and weakest crewmember can still launch the raft.

Do not pack your primary EPIRB inside the liferaft. Abandoning ship is not the only time you or your crew may need to set off the EPIRB, and it would be extremely awkward to have to inflate your liferaft to operate the beacon. But a second EPIRB packed inside the liferaft is an excellent idea. An EPIRB is the single most important item of survival equipment that you can have in your liferaft to communicate with the world. Surviving is necessary, but the ultimate aim is to be rescued quickly.

▶ Servicing Your Liferaft

Servicing is expensive but necessary, and extending the period between services only makes it more likely that the raft will require more expensive repairs later, or even be condemned early. Servicing should be undertaken for three reasons:

- To replace dated items like medicines, flares, batteries and water.

- To inspect for water damage and make sure the inflation cylinder is full.
- To check the raft for wear, particularly at the folds.

Service intervals of liferafts vary enormously so set up a calendar alert to ensure the raft is taken ashore to a service agent at the correct time. Always choose a centre that will allow you and your crew to be present so you can watch as your raft is opened. This may be the only chance you ever get to see your raft and personally check its equipment before you need to use it.

▶ Renting a Raft

If you normally sail close to the coast, buying a liferaft may seem an unnecessary expense for your annual holiday trip further afield or for an offshore race. Renting a liferaft has become a very popular option and it is possible to rent for as short a time as a weekend, or for as long as a year or more. The same care must be taken with choosing a rented liferaft as with a purchased model. Ensure you know exactly what the emergency pack contains so you know how much you need to pack in your grab bag to supplement it. Always check that the rental raft was serviced immediately prior to your hiring, so you know it is in good condition and contains everything listed.

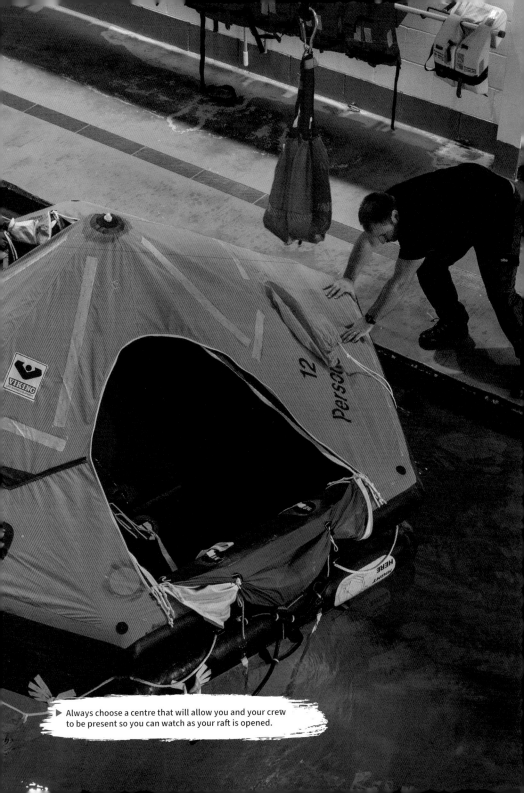

▶ Always choose a centre that will allow you and your crew to be present so you can watch as your raft is opened.

3 YOUR GRAB BAG AND ITS CONTENTS

To decide what to pack in your grab bag you must first answer a few questions about your proposed trip:
- *What is contained in my liferaft?*
- *What is the quality of that equipment?*
- *Where will the boat be sailing?*
- *What is the maximum crew number aboard?*

Perhaps a grab bag is best viewed as life insurance, with you and your crew as the immediate beneficiaries. It's just a matter of deciding on the premium you are willing to pay for the lives of yourself and your crew. Sadly, assembling a comprehensive grab bag will not be cheap. Some items will last almost forever, and others will need to be replaced at regular intervals.

▶ Choosing a Container

CHOOSING THE RIGHT container for your grab bag is somewhat of a chicken and egg situation. Do you decide what you want when you abandon ship and choose a bag to fit it all? Or do you select the bag to fit the stowage position you have in mind, then and see how much you can fit in?

A soft dry bag is easier to handle and live with in a liferaft, but a rigid and buoyant waterproof box may be towed to provide more space.

There are certain common properties that every grab bag should have, regardless of how large or small: Every grab bag should be:
- Ideally brightly coloured, waterproof and able to float.
- Clearly marked with the name of your yacht and the words 'GRAB BAG'.
- Striped with reflective tape (such as T-ISS SolasFlex Retro Reflective Tape) designed for the marine environment and lifesaving appliances.
- Fitted with a lanyard to attach it to the liferaft.

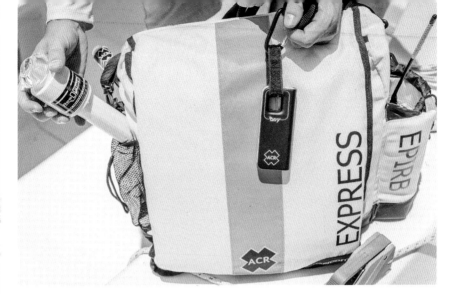

▶ A soft dry bag is easier to handle and live with in a liferaft.

- Duplicated to match the number of liferafts carried.

Inside the bag:

- Shape a domestic cutting board to fit the base to reinforce the bottom of a soft bag and prevent sagging. This will be useful for cutting things while in the raft.
- Use closed-cell foam for cushioning and extra flotation.
- Seal individual items inside waterproof bags.
- Use a vacuum-bagging machine to seal bags and reduce size to a minimum.
- Store small items in waterproof boxes, or jars with secure lids
- List the contents of all sealed items on the outside using a waterproof marker.
- Include any equipment instructions on waterproof paper.
- Attach a lanyard to everything possible to prevent loss, especially in rough weather.

- Cover anything with a sharp point that could puncture your raft, eg, tip of gaff.

Once the bag is chosen and filled, check it will still float. Stow the bag on deck or close by, ideally in the cockpit on a sailboat or the wheelhouse on a motorboat.

Every crewmember must know exactly where the grab bag lives and what it contains. They should also be able to handle the fully laden bag (if necessary, consider splitting the load into two smaller bags).

Whatever you decide it will probably be a compromise – the bag from the movie *Mary Poppins* would be perfect as it was much bigger inside than out. Try to pack the bag so that items likely to be needed first, like the maintenance and protection equipment, are at the top. If you have decided to split the load into two bags and cannot stow them both in an ideal spot, you will have to prioritise or split items. An empty spare bag, kept handy, is a good idea to use for stowing some of your Last-minute Grabs.

▶ What to Pack in Your Grab Bag

The rest of this chapter details suggested items to pack in your grab bag. These have been divided into a series of categories:

- Search and Rescue
- Maintenance and Protection
- Medical
- Food and Drink
- Survival and Morale
- Personal
- Miscellaneous
- Last-minute Grabs

With the exception of Last-minute Grabs, the categories are in order of priority, but the items listed within are purely in alphabetical order.

Items marked with an asterisk* are those you would find in most comprehensive standard emergency liferaft pack, such as SOLAS 'A'.

▶ Search and Rescue Equipment

This category almost ties for first place with Maintenance and Protection, but because achieving rescue is what you want more than anything else, it wins by a short head. A liferaft is extremely difficult to spot especially in rough seas. The more you can do in your liferaft to attract attention, and the more methods of signalling you have available, the more likely it is that someone will come

to your aid. The more items you have in this category, the less you should need of other categories.

EPIRB

This device is probably **the most important piece of equipment that you can take in a liferaft**. Even though you may already have made contact by radio, your EPIRB will help the Search and Rescue authorities (SAR) home in on your position. Carrying an EPIRB with built-in GPS will make up for a great many other deficiencies your grab bag might suffer from, and it will almost certainly ensure you spend hours in a liferaft rather than weeks. The only thing better than an EPIRB when you need it, is a second EPIRB as a backup!

There are two types of EPIRB to consider:

Category I – will automatically deploy and activate by means of a hydrostatic release if the EPIRB sinks below 1–3m (3–10ft). These are required aboard GMDSS-compliant vessels. The unit can also be operated manually.

Category II – manual operation only. The unit must be removed from its housing and plunged into water, or the power button must be pressed.

For non-GMDSS-compliant boats, choosing between the categories is difficult, even without considering the financial factor. At first glance an automatic Category I EPIRB looks best, but:

- It is more expensive.
- It must be mounted on deck and clear of obstacles, so it can float free.
- It must not be underwater while sailing, as this could cause false activation.

- Sinking involving a dismasting could obscure the unit and prevent it ever floating free.

With these thoughts in mind, and especially if you only purchase one unit, a good choice might be:

- Category II EPIRB in the top of your grab bag on a sailing yacht.
- Category I EPIRB aboard a motor yacht.
- But best of all: on any yacht, mount a Category I EPIRB on deck, pack a Category II in your grab bag and have everyone wear PLBs.

Whichever choice you make, ensure the EPIRB is handy and that all crewmembers know where it is and how it works. Make sure it is marked with your yacht's name, like all major safety items, in case it becomes separated from your vessel or liferaft. Lost but marked items can give rescuers valuable information using known drift rates and the vessel's identity.

It cannot be emphasised strongly enough how important it is to **register every EPIRB, including personal EPIRBS** (Note: AIS units cannot be registered):

- Fill in and send off the registration card that comes with the beacon.
- If you have lost the card, details of where to register are in Sources of Supplies and Information in the Appendix.

When an EPIRB is activated these details enable the Coastguard authorities to telephone your listed emergency contact. Your shoreside contact can:

- Provide valuable information to help confirm your possible position.

- Rule out the possibility of a false alarm, which sadly still accounts for eight out of nine transmissions.
- Give important extra information from your Voyage Details Plan (see Appendix).

Once an EPIRB is purchased there is no additional cost apart from replacing the battery, which will usually last for years if unused. There is no subscription cost for the emergency tracking system.

Flares/pyrotechnics

Flares, also called pyrotechnics, are recognised distress signals designed to alert people that you are in trouble and provide a location signal for would-be rescuers to home in on. Ensure that the flares you choose meet SOLAS recommendations. There are other flares on the market that do not meet that standard of burn time or brightness, but if you are in distress you will want all the signalling power you can get. Beware of cheap pyrotechnics, they can cause accidents.

An in-date flare kit, stored in a waterproof container where it can be quickly located in an emergency, should be part of every yacht's equipment no matter where you sail. This flare container should be included on your Last-minute Grab List and spare out-of-date flares can also be included in your grab bag. Add extra flares to your grab bag if your liferaft emergency pack is deficient or, better still, have them packed inside the liferaft.

Pyrotechnics can, by their very nature, be considered dangerous when handled incorrectly. It pays to familiarise yourself with their safe operation before you need to use them in an emergency.

Training courses that offer hands-on firing experience are a good way of gaining such familiarisation.

Flares – orange smoke*

SOLAS specification buoyant smoke signals burn for not less than three minutes, and will not ignite oil or fuel. They should be carried for all offshore passages. If you never intend to sail far from shore, handheld orange flares, which burn for about one minute, may be sufficient.

Flares – red handheld*

SOLAS specification red handheld flares have a minimum burning period of one minute and a luminous intensity of 15,000 candela; nothing less should be carried. A minimum of three should be carried aboard all yachts and three packed in every liferaft or grab bag.

Flares – red parachute*

SOLAS specification red parachute flares, with self-container launchers, reach 300m (1,000ft) in altitude and burn for a minimum of 40 seconds. Pack plenty for any trip to sea; they can attract attention at great distances, including ships that are over your horizon.

Flares – white parachute

Not an emergency signal as such, but a white parachute flare is excellent for lighting an area in an emergency.

LED flares

Modern, battery-powered, electronic LED 'flares' are now available. They are not comparable to a pyrotechnic flare in power or visibility, and they are not approved by the authorities, but they are much safer than a conventional flare and have a longer burn time. One would make a useful addition, but not a replacement, for pyrotechnics in any grab bag.

Flashlight/torch*

A waterproof model to be used for signalling is included in all standard liferaft emergency packs, along with a spare bulb and batteries. Even a very small flashlight is extremely effective at night for signalling.

Some liferafts have no internal light, so pack a flashlight near the top of your grab bag in case you have to abandon ship at night.

Diving lights are a good choice as they must be waterproof. A floating model is a bonus; make sure you can fit a lanyard. A waterproof hands-free headtorch light is a plus.

Ensure, if possible, that all flashlights use the same size batteries and pack plenty of spares. Stock rotate all batteries with yacht's regular supply and include the grab bag flashlights on the list of items to check before a passage. Flashlights

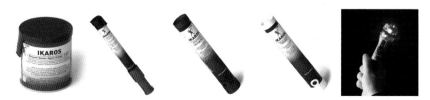

▶ Flares (from left) include orange smoke, red handheld, red parachute, white parachute and LED.

with rechargeable batteries should also be checked.

Kite

A highly visible kite attracts attention and helps rescuers pinpoint your location, plus it's fun to fly!

PLB

The skipper of any yacht making an offshore passage or sailing in rough weather should ensure each member of crew is wearing a PLB on deck. It is the same as a lifejacket – it makes good sense. Storing spare PLBs not currently in use or adding an extra one to the grab bag is a good idea.

Finally, there is little point in having a PLB and it not being registered. Before setting off on a voyage, ensure each unit is registered and the emergency contact details are up to date. If the emergency contact of any unit is not the shoreside contact, make sure that person also knows what voyage is planned and let them know when the yacht arrives at the destination.

Radar reflector*

Rafts do not reflect radar waves well and, unfortunately, it is hard to get a reflector high enough to be effective, especially in a big sea. Even if your emergency pack includes a reflector seriously consider purchasing an AIS SART. If money is very tight a standard radar reflector is better than nothing.

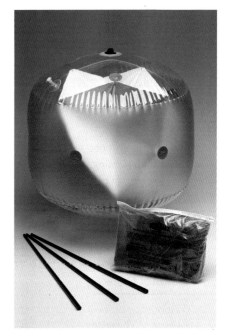

▶ An Echomax inflatable ball reflector.

Rescue line and quoit*

This should be included in every liferaft, with not less than 30m (100ft) of buoyant line and fastened to the raft. It is designed to throw from the liferaft to a survivor in the water, to assist them reaching the raft.

SART*

A Search and Rescue Transponder (SART), also called a Radar Transponder, is an extremely valuable addition to your EPIRB:

• It returns a magnified, directional, unmistakable, emergency image to any marine radar.

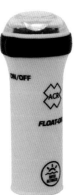

▶ An ACR float.

- The signal is received by any marine radar operating within range.
- Most commercial vessels and larger yachts have radar.
- The distinctive signal is easily recognised and much easier to spot than the single echo from a radar reflector.
- It does not require specialised equipment for homing.
- The radar can then be used to guide the rescue craft to the exact location of the SART.
- It is required aboard any vessel that is GMDSS-compliant.

SOLAS signal table*

A waterproof copy of the illustrated table of SOLAS No 2 Lifesaving Signals (also on page 136) should be included in every liferaft. These visual signals are used between shore stations in the UK and ships in distress.

Signal mirror*

Also known as a heliograph, this is the most basic and probably cheapest all-round signalling device for use on land or sea. Its advantages include:

- It is compact and simple to use.
- Any shiny object can be used.
- A purpose-made mirror is brighter and easier to aim.
- Buoyant waterproof models are designed for marine use. Make

sure the instructions for use are on waterproof paper.

- It is used to reflect the sun's ray towards rescue personnel.
- It can be used to transmit Morse code, but a simple flash is easier to send.
- In normal sunlight the flash can be seen from at least 10 miles (16km).
- A signal mirror will take up little room in your grab bag.
- The more you have, the better. Pack one for each crewmember.
- With two mirrors you can sweep the horizon.

Strobe light

Rapidly flashing strobe lights stand out in open water. They are blindingly bright at close range, but further away are less obvious because the light is dispersed rather than directed. Its major advantage is that it can operate unattended. However, directed light from even a very small flashlight is much more visible and at a far greater distance than a strobe. If your raft is not already fitted with one, attach a strobe from your grab bag to the outside of the liferaft at night for added visibility.

Survival craft radio

Survival craft aboard GMDSS-compliant vessels must carry a waterproof handheld VHF. It makes sense yachts should carry them even though they may not need to be compliant. Where money was no object, the ultimate grab bag would

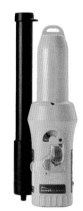

▶ A Radar Transponder is an extremely valuable addition to your EPIRB.

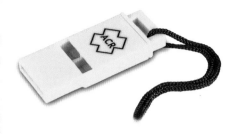

▶ A whistle assists with location in the water.

include one of these or, at the very least, a less powerful waterproof and buoyant handheld VHF capable of transmitting on at least three channels viz 3, 6 and 16.

Whistle*

A whistle will not attract the attention of a ship or passing aeroplane, but it can help anyone in the water to locate the liferaft. They are cheap and small, so pack a couple of powerful ones. In theory, everyone in the liferaft should be carrying one, attached to their lifejacket.

▶ Maintenance and Protection

The better the quality of your liferaft, the fewer of these items you should need to use. Unfortunately, the longer you must survive in the raft, the more items you will need. An ocean grab bag and liferaft should include at least one of every item here, whereas a yacht never venturing far from shore can reduce this list.

Bailer*

Every liferaft should come with a bailer, though their quality may be doubtful.

Sadly, your liferaft is unlikely to stay dry and you will be doing a lot of bailing. A plastic dinghy bailer with a handle is cheap enough, so pack a couple. Small items can be packed inside them, so they shouldn't take up too much room. If you have enough space, include a hand pump type as well; it will remove large quantities of water quickly and easily.

Bucket

A bucket has many uses from additional bailer to makeshift privy. A collapsible model or a folding bowl will fit inside a grab bag. Otherwise, pack a small child's seaside bucket. Add the location of the ship's buckets used for washing down etc, to your Last-minute Grabs list and use them as carrying containers at abandon ship time.

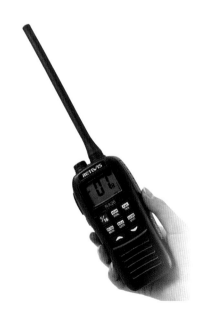

▶ A handheld VHF is capable of transmitting on at least three channels.

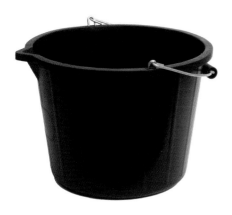
▶ A bucket has many uses.

Chemical heat pack

Hand and body chemical heat packs can provide welcome warmth; the beginnings of hypothermia can set in after a very short time in almost any waters. Hand warming packs can give up to 10 hours of gentle warmth, with larger body packs claiming to offer 20+ hours. The colder the conditions you will be sailing in, the more of these you should include in your grab bag.

Diving mask/swimming goggles

If you need to swim under the raft to carry out any repairs, you will be very grateful that you packed either a diving mask or a pair of swimming goggles. They can also be used by the lookout as protection against driving rain or heavy seas.

Inflatable cushions

Some sort of inflatable cushion or mattress will make life very much more comfortable, especially if your liferaft has no additional insulated floor, either inflatable or foam. It will help to keep you above the water that inevitably finds its way into a raft.

Light sticks

Many rafts have no light or, where fitted, it cannot be turned off. Whatever your liferaft has it will not last long, and you will need some other form of interior light at night. Chemical light sticks are cheap to buy and unaffected by the marine environment, giving a gentle light that can last all night. However, they are easy to accidentally activate and must be packed very carefully.

Battery-operated waterproof light sticks, sold in dive shops, are much longer lasting and can be switched on and off. But they are vulnerable in the marine environment, like all electrical items.

Pack a selection of chemical and battery-operated models for the best of both worlds.

Paddles*

A pair of paddles should be included in every liferaft, to assist with moving away from the mother ship. Not all paddles are full-sized or buoyant. One liferaft manufacturer, for example, supplies hand paddles made of fabric! It is unlikely that you will be paddling far in most liferafts though. Certainly, a circular raft is hard to move in a particular direction with paddles alone.

Pump*

A bellows or hand pump should be part of every liferaft equipment bag for topping up the buoyancy chambers, but the quality is often miserable. It should be in one piece, ready for use without any assembling; if yours is not, pack one that is in your grab bag. It is a vital piece of equipment for long time survival in a liferaft; in fact, a spare one is a very good idea for an ocean grab bag. An inflatable dinghy pump may be an option, used with an adapter, but make sure it isn't designed for foot use only. Check with your liferaft supplier that any pump you choose will work with your raft.

Repair kit*

Liferafts all come with a repair kit of some kind, but not necessarily a useful one, so check it carefully. It's all too common to find the kit consists of patches and glue that require a clean and dry surface, almost inconceivable in a liferaft! Make

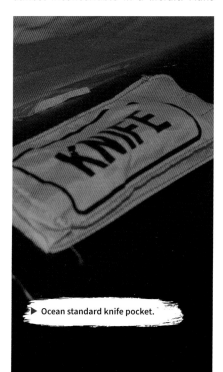

► Ocean standard knife pocket.

up your own kit, with equipment that is suitable for your liferaft, and pack it near the top of your grab bag with the following:

- Spare canopy and raft material.
- Glue that will work in a wet and salty environment.
- Varity of needles, including sail repair needles, some waxed thread and sewing awl.
- Assorted sized leak stopper plugs for a temporary repair.
- Assorted sized hose clamps to tighten the raft material around a plug.
- Assorted sized raft repair clamps. These are the easiest way to repair a hole with an airtight seal.
- Spare plugs for pressure release and topping up valves.

Rope

Pack a large assortment of long lengths of rope and twine in your grab bag to use as lashings, lanyards and general improvisation.

Safety knife*

This has a blunt tipped blade supposedly incapable of harming the raft or a person. It is included with a liferaft, stored near the entrance, to cut the painter if necessary. A knife meeting SOLAS specifications will have a buoyant handle. This knife is not likely to be much use for any serious cutting and you will need to supplement it (see page 45).

Sail repair tape

Heavy-duty sail tape is designed for the salt environment and is very useful for quick repairs and improvisations. This makes a valuable addition to the more multipurpose elephant tape included under Miscellaneous.

Sea anchor*

Also called a drogue, the purpose of the sea anchor is to reduce the drift rate of the liferaft and to reduce the risk of capsize. All liferafts include a sea anchor, but its quality and effectiveness may vary. If your raft is not to SOLAS standard, consider including one in the grab bag and upgrade your liferaft sea anchor at the next service.

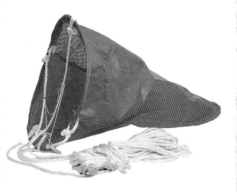

▶ A sea anchor helps to reduce a liferaft's drift rate.

A sea anchor has an additional use, to help the paddles move a circular liferaft in a particular direction. Unfortunately, they are all too easy to lose in rough weather.

- Every liferaft has one.
- A self-deploying version attached to the liferaft is the best.
- Include at least one spare in your grab bag, unless you have a SOLAS emergency liferaft pack.
- Ensure there is a minimum of 15m (49ft) of attachment line with swivels at each end to help prevent fouling.

Sponges

Sponges are cheap and included in many liferaft packs. SOLAS packs include two, while the 1998 Sydney–Hobart Race Coroner recommended one per person. In theory, they are for drying and mopping up residual water from the floor of the raft. They are also very useful for collecting condensation from the inside of the canopy to drink, so keep at least one free of salt water for this purpose. Very absorbent small sponges, that require only one hand to squeeze out, are best.

Sunscreen

Sunscreen can provide important protection against the misery of sunburn when you are on the water. It is very easy to underestimate the power of the sun, even on an overcast day, to burn human skin. This is especially true in the tropics but a bright day in the high latitudes can burn, too. Pack high SPF waterproof sunscreen for face and body, plus an SPF 30 product for lips, no matter how close to shore you sail. Make a note of the expiry dates and replace as necessary – out of date sunscreen will not be as effective.

Thermal protective aid*

A space blanket is not a substitute for a thermal protective aid (TPA); it is unsuitable for liferaft use. Instead, use a thermal protective aid. This is a special bag designed to fully enclose a person, covering from head to toe and always including a hood.

It keeps a survivor warm by reflecting back the body heat and is a lifesaving piece of kit in the treatment of hypothermia.

Body-shaped models feature arms and legs, allowing various activities without removing the TPA. A bag shape is more efficient at retaining heat and could accommodate two people for re-warming. The outer edges are sealed, except the cuffs of arms, and it is impermeable up to the zip or Velcro. Even in a partly water-filled liferaft, your feet will remain dry.

Make sure you pack one for every crewmember, no matter how little else you pack in your grab bag; ideally a selection of the two shape types.

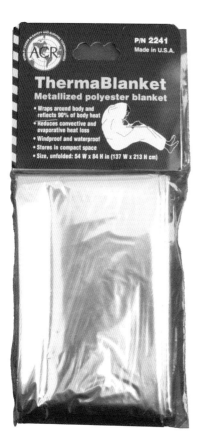

▶ A thermal reflective aid reflects back body heat.

Umbrella

This might seem a strange item to include in your grab bag, and those of Italian extraction may consider it very unlucky, but it can be very useful:

- It is light and cheap.
- It can be used by the liferaft lookout as a sunshade or for rain cover.
- If your raft lacks a canopy, include one per person to provide valuable shade.
- It can act as a rainwater catcher.

Watch hat

To give the watchkeeper a measure of comfort, pack a hat to protect against sun or cold, depending upon your sailing area. If your liferaft is a basic inshore model, without a canopy, include a hat for every crewmember.

▶ Medical

The further you are sailing the more of the following items you should add to your grab bag.

Anti-seasickness tablets*

Even if you are one of those lucky people who never suffers from *mal de mer*, you probably will in a liferaft for the following reasons:

- Abandoning ship more often occurs in rough weather than calm conditions.
- A survival craft is very small and generally tightly enclosed.
- Even if you don't feel sick to start with, seeing someone else ill, right next to you, is very hard on even the strongest stomach.

Seasickness causes the loss of valuable fluids that may be very difficult to replace in a raft and can lead to serious dehydration. It also makes you more prone to hypothermia and this can eventually kill you.

There are many different anti-seasickness preparations available over the counter, pack ones that work for you and your crew, and view any in your liferaft pack as extra. Include prescription anti-emetic drugs in your first aid kit.

Enema kit

The MCA issues a list of medical supplies that must be carried by various classes of vessels, which is a valuable guide for any yacht planning to make an ocean passage. An enema kit, or rectal drip, is on this list to rehydrate a patient unable to take liquids orally. It is a valuable piece of equipment for severe seasickness, when the patient is unable to retain anything taken by mouth and dehydration becomes a major problem. This could happen in a liferaft. Another use for an enema kit is for re-hydration if your water supply is unpalatable. However, this is not a method of ingesting seawater.

First aid kit*

British SOLAS specified liferaft packs must include a Category C first aid kit packed in a sealed re-useable container, together with first aid instructions printed on waterproof paper. The Category C medical supplies are listed on pages 40–1. If your liferaft kit does not include this, or its equivalent, consider having a Category

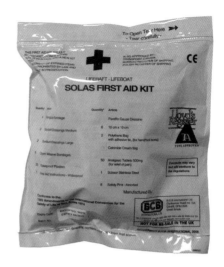

▶ Category C first aid kits are packed in a sealed, re-usable container.

C kit packed into your liferaft or included in your grab bag.

First aid outfits supplied inside liferafts are packed in durable, damp-proof and effectively sealed containers, capable of being closed tightly after use. They must bear on the outside an itemised list of the contents and their date of expiry.

Your Last-minute Grabs list should include the yacht's medical kit packed in a waterproof container. In case it is impossible to grab the yacht's kit, particularly the prescription drugs, in time, consider adding a few duplicate items to your grab bag, especially when sailing offshore:

- Prescription topical anti-bacterial ointment, as germs breed quickly in a liferaft.
- Aspirin as a first aid treatment for heart attacks. Aspirin helps to thin the blood and improves blood flow to

the heart. Chewing and then swallowing a tablet of aspirin (ideally 300mg), may help as a first aid treatment as long as the person having a heart attack is not allergic to aspirin.

- Transparent waterproof and breathable adhesive bandages, which if put on dry skin will stay in place and seal a wound even in water.

- Prescription anti-emetic in suppository or injectable form for severe seasickness.
- Inflatable splints for broken limbs.

A comprehensive medical kit is useless without some knowledge and training. At least two members of the crew should know what to do in a medical emergency, and ideally everyone should have a basic

LIFERAFT FIRST AID KIT
(Category C Medical Supplies)

Ref No.	Statutory treatment requirements	Recommended medicine and dosage strength representing best practice	Quantity
1	**Cardio vascular**		
(b)	Anti-angina preparations *For suspected heart attack or heart pain*	Glyceryl Trinitrate Spray 400 micrograms/metered 200 dose aerosol or transdermal patches 5mg x 2	1 unit
(d)	Anti-haemorrhagics (anti-bleeding) (including uterotonics if there are women with potential for child bearing)	i) Phytomenadione (Vitamin K1) 10mg in 1ml ampoule *paediatric injection Anti-haemorrhage for new born babies*	1
		ii) Ergometrine Maleate 500mg inj. Oxytocin 5 units in 1ml ampoule *For use immediately after delivery of baby or for bleeding after miscarriage*	1
2	**Gastro intestinal system**		
(b)	Anti-emetics (anti-sickness)	Hyoscine hydrobromide 0.3mg tabs	60
(d)	Anti-diarrhoeals	Codeine phosphate 30mg tabs (also painkiller)	20
3	**Analgesics and anti-spasmodics**		
(a)	Analgesics Painkillers	i) Paracetamol *Mild to moderate pain*	50
		ii) Codeine phosphate (see 2d) *Moderate to severe pain*	Use 2(d)
4	**Nervous system**		
(c)	Seasickness remedies	Hyoscine hydrobromide (see 2b)	Use 2(b)
9	**Medicines for external use**		
(a)	Skin medicine		
	– Antisepœtic solutions	100ml solution or pre-impregnated wipes containing 0.015% w/v chlorhexidine and 0.15% w/v cetrimide	1 bottle or 1 pack wipes
	– Burn preparations	Cetrimide cream 50g tube	1

LIFERAFT FIRST AID KIT
(Category C Medical Supplies)

MEDICAL EQUIPMENT

Ref No.	Statutory treatment requirements	Recommended specification	Quantity
1	**Resuscitation equipment**		
	Mask for mouth-to-mouth resuscitation	Laerdal pocket mask or similar	1
2	**Dressing and suturing equipment**		
	Adhesive elastic bandage	Adhesive elastic bandage 7.5cm x 4m	1
	Disposable polyethylene gloves	Large size	5prs
	Adhesive dressings	Assorted, sterile	20
	Sterile compression bandages and unmedicated dressings	No. 13 Medium, 10 x 8cm No. 14 Large, 13 x 9cm No. 15 Extra large, 28 x 17.5cm	6 2 2
	Adhesive sutures or zinc oxide bandages	75mm adhesive suture strips	6
	Sterile gauze compresses	Packet containing 5 sterile gauze pads size 7.5 x 7.5cm	1
	Recommended additional item		
	Scissors	Stainless steel or sterile disposable	1pr
	Calico triangular bandages	About 90 x 127cm	4
	Medium safety pins, rustless		6
	Sterile paraffin gauze dressings		10
	Plastic burn bags		1

The Reference Number (Ref No.) refers to the number allocated to the medicine or equipment in MSN 1676(M)

knowledge, especially of resuscitation and CPR.

Petroleum jelly

It is not only a valuable medical addition, but can also be used for protecting metal. It is an extremely versatile product for lubrication.

▶ Seasickness bags are incredibly useful.

Seasickness bags*

It is bad enough being seasick, but having nothing to be sick into makes your misery total. Pack a roll or two of biodegradable dog poo bags, or other cheap plastic bags, in your grab bag. These are much better than the airline style paper bags, which could disintegrate if the liferaft is very wet.

Sunburn cream

It's hard to avoid getting sunburned without protection from the sun, especially in the tropics on deceptively overcast days. Pack at least one tube, (more for large crews); creams that include aloe are very good for treating sunburn.

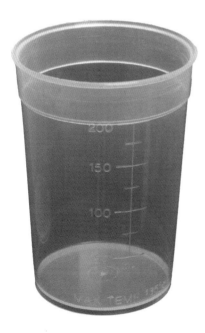

▶ A graduated drinking cup.

▶ Food and drink

Food and water are unnecessary in the short term. If you are sailing inshore in busy waters, carrying an EPIRB, a portable VHF or a telephone, you probably do not need any of the items in this list. On the other hand, if you are planning to sail further afield or you have skimped on the equipment in the Search and Research category, then rescue may be delayed. Even with plenty of signalling equipment when crossing oceans or sailing far off normal shipping routes, help may be some time in arriving. In the medium term you will need water and in the long-term food, plus a means of gathering both yourself.

Can opener*

A can opener is included in all liferaft packs, even those that do not contain water and food in tins. You and your crew should all be wearing a multipurpose tool or folding knife, making this item unnecessary, but, for security, include at least one can opener in your grab bag to undo any tins you might grab from the galley as you abandon ship.

Containers

Use various sizes of containers, with watertight lids, to pack items in your grab bag. The containers can serve double duty as water collectors or bailers. Also include collapsible water carriers to store collected or made water, and to hold the water from the liferaft water packs.

Cutlery

For a small amount of money and space, a few sets of bamboo or other eco picnic cutlery make everyone feel more civilised.

Cutting board

Using a cutting board in the bottom of your grab bag to make it firm and easier to handle was discussed earlier. Though it is possible to improvise using some types of paddles supplied in a liferaft, others, such as the canvas style, would be hopeless. If you want to fillet a fish for example, a board is invaluable. A polyethylene antibacterial kitchen chopping board is ideal, as water will not hurt it. If space is at a premium, choose a small 'backpackers' chopping board instead.

Drinking cups*

Liferaft packs that include water also include a graduated drinking cup to fairly divide up the water. Add light bamboo or eco picnic cups, for example, to your grab bag so you can toast each other with a cocktail hour water ration! They can serve double functions as bailers or water catchers.

Drinking water*

SOLAS 'A', 'B' and 24-hour plus liferaft packs contain 1.5l (0.4 gallons) of water per person, while others allow 0.5l (0.1 gallons). If you are planning to undertake an ocean passage, ensure your liferaft contains at least 0.5l (0.1 gallons) per person; if this is impossible, then pack water into your grab bag. Do this in addition to any portable watermaker

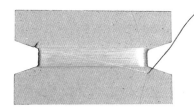
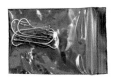

▶ A basic fishing kit includes line and hooks.

you carry. Before any long passage, store as many large plastic bottles as you have room for, 80 per cent full of water. Alternatively, empty 20 per cent from large bottles of mineral water and reseal. Store these bottles on deck, as near to your grab bag or liferaft as possible. Tied together with a floating line, these partially filled bottles will float in seawater and can be towed behind the raft to free up space inside.

Fishing kit*

A rather basic fishing kit is included in SOLAS 'A' liferaft packs and usually comprises of a line and six hooks. No bait is supplied, and since fish should not be eaten without a plentiful supply of water (see Chapter 7), the inclusion of fishing gear may be questionable, especially if all you have in the way of drinking water is the 0.5l (0.1 gallons) supplied in non-SOLAS liferaft packs. So, why have fishing equipment? Four good reasons:

- The rescue authorities may have been alerted, but they still have to reach you.

- Long-term survival in a liferaft depends on obtaining food as well as water.
- Fishing helps pass the time and can improve morale.
- The equipment can be put to another use such as repairing the liferaft.

Your grab bag should include a fishing kit with tackle to catch small to medium fish, not large game fish! They would be impossible to land safely in a vulnerable liferaft. Unless you are a fishing expert, visit a specialist shop and ask for help in packing a small, but comprehensive, kit. Make sure everything is of the highest quality and anything metal is, if possible, made from stainless steel to prevent serious rusting as it sits in your grab bag. The kit should include:

- 100m (300ft) light fishing line.
- Two small hand winders; if they are too big for your bag consider a kite winder.
- Wire leaders with clip-on swivels.
- Clip-on swivels.
- Assorted sinkers.
- Plentiful supply of assorted hooks.
- Various lures.
- Small gaff or net to help land fish.
- Waterproof instruction booklet.

Food rations

Liferaft packs contain approximately three days' worth of food when operating in mild or warm weather. In cold weather and cold waters, where more energy and thus food, is required to keep warm, this ration will not last as long. Liferaft survival rations are specially designed for consumption with minimal water and so they are high in carbohydrates, and low in protein (which requires more water for digestion/elimination). Buy

this special survival food to pack in your grab bag, particularly if your liferaft does not include any or only a small amount. These foods may not taste great, but they are better than anything else you can buy. *Do not pack the dehydrated food found in outdoor stores as, like the food you are likely to catch, it requires much more water.* Extra items to pack should be high in carbohydrates and sugar, but low in protein:

- Boiled sweets (hard candy).
- Chocolate.
- Dried fruit.
- Energy bars.
- Glucose tablets.
- Tinned fruit.
- Tinned sweetened milk.

Funnel

Useful to transfer water between containers and ensures not a drop is wasted.

Gloves

A couple of pairs of thick gloves, either leather or man-made material, with non-slip palms, are invaluable to protect hands, especially when fishing.

Multivitamin tablets

For long-term liferaft survival, include 30 days' supply per person of chewable multivitamin tablets.

Solar still

Sun, salt water and a solar still can produce fresh drinking water. On land, a still is fairly easy to construct but, at sea, this might only be feasible with flat, calm conditions. One commercially produced version of a solar still designed to work at sea is the inflatable Aquamate Solar Still which, in theory, can make between 0.5–2l (0.1–0.5 gallons) of water a day.

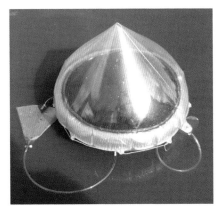

▶ A solar still can produce fresh drinking water.

Watermaker

A reverse osmosis watermaker is the most reliable way of making drinking water out of salt water, and handheld units are included in some liferafts as part of the standard equipment. Along with your EPIRBs, this is the most important item

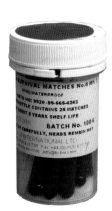

▶ A pocket-sized watertight container of matches can prove invaluable in the event that you make landfall.

you can pack in a grab bag. There are, at present, only two choices of small manual watermakers on the market, both made by Katadyn in Switzerland:
- Survivor 06 – can make just over 1l (0.25 gallons) of fresh water per hour.
- Survivor 35 –the larger version, can make 5.5l (1.5 gallons) per hour. This model is preferable for crews of eight or more.

Neither are cheap, but then nor is your life or that of your crew.

▶ Survival and Morale

The items in this category are a mixture of those required to live for a long period in the liferaft and those that may be needed at any time, plus a few items designed to keep everyone entertained.

Charts

Ship routeing, current and wind charts are not so much for navigation, which is very difficult in an inflatable liferaft, but should be included with morale in mind. Used with your compass, they will give you an idea of where you are drifting, possible landfalls and sources of rescue. If your charts are not on waterproof paper, laminate them.

Compass

Pack a small plastic compass to keep track of how you are drifting, or for use if you reach the shore.

Knife

Include a large non-ferrous, sturdy, fixed-blade knife In your grab bag. A dive knife

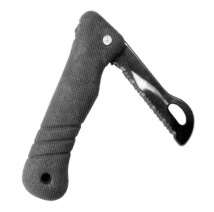

▶ A good folding knife is incredibly useful.

may be suitable, but some survivalists recommend avoiding double-edged knives. Pack the knife blade covered in petroleum jelly inside a plastic sheaf, to prevent it from rusting while it sits in your grab bag.

Knife sharpener

A stone or ceramic sharpener is best as it will not be adversely affected by salt water.

Land survival book

The Collins Gem SAS Survival Book, for example, is very comprehensive yet small enough to fit into a corner of your grab bag. If you make your own way ashore in a desolate part of the world, it will be an invaluable guide to living off the land. Pack it inside at least two sealed plastic bags to keep it dry until you reach land.

Land survival kit

Pack a few things for landfall, either a ready-made set or select your own small items. Make sure they are packed in a pocket-sized watertight container

and include firelighters, matches, a magnifying glass, water purification tablets, a wire saw and a snare.

Lighter

A windproof refillable lighter (with spare butane) will be useful for sealing things like polypropylene rope in the liferaft, as well as starting a fire ashore.

Multipurpose tool

Everyone aboard a yacht should carry their own folding knife, but also pack into the grab bag at least one multipurpose tool. Choose one with a good assortment of extras such as pliers, bottle opener, scissors, screwdrivers, wire cutter, serrated knife, file, awl/punch etc. Use petroleum jelly to coat the blades etc and, if possible, vacuum seal the tool to prevent rusting.

Pack of cards

A pack of waterproof playing cards is ideal to while away the hours of waiting.

Pens and pencils

Pack a few writing instruments that work on waterproof paper; you'll need to keep score of that poker game.

Scissors

Include a strong pair of kitchen scissors in your grab bag. These are extremely useful, especially when conditions are too rough to use a knife safely. Pack the scissors with the blades coated in petroleum jelly.

Solar chargers/battery bank

Portable phones, VHFs and even music players brought with you will all need to be recharged. Be prepared by packing a portable solar panel, typically marketed for backpacking, hiking or camping. We strongly recommend pairing this with a separate external USB battery bank so that you do not ruin your device batteries by baking them in the sun during a charge cycle.

Survival Instructions*

Every liferaft should come with some basic instructions about survival. Better still, seal a copy of this book inside a couple of plastic bags and pack it away inside your grab bag. Alternatively, remove and laminate pages you wish to take with you.

Towels

Pack a couple of microfibre towels, well-sealed against water. They can be used in many ways for repairs and improvisations, such as a pad to stop bleeding, protecting against chafe, cleaning, collecting water, as well as the obvious: drying yourself.

Waterproof paper notebook

It is important you keep a log in a liferaft, as a memory aid and for morale. Who knows, you may write a book with first-hand experience that rivals this one! Make sure any paper you pack is waterproof.

▶ *Personal*

Contact lens kit

If any of the crew needs to wear contact lenses, include the maintenance kit or daily wear lenses as appropriate. Make sure you also include a pair of prescription glasses for any contact lens wearer, as it may be impossible for them to keep wearing the lenses and they may not be wearing them when abandoning ship.

Condoms

Pack some away! If not for the manufacturer's intended use, then because they make excellent water storage devices.

Credit card

Duplicate or spare credit/debit cards can ease things when you reach shore, especially in a foreign country. Ensure the card is the type that will enable you to get a cash advance from a bank, ATM or cash point machine.

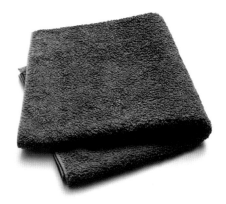

▶ Towels may have many different uses.

47

Money

Sometimes nothing but cash will do, so include some in your grab bag; how much is up to you. If you are sailing locally only, include the currency of the country, in small denominations. Those travelling further afield should include US dollars, which are widely accepted.

Personal hygiene items

Toothbrush, toothpaste and some moist towelettes are a great morale booster, plus help to keep you healthy. Brushing their teeth makes most people feel much better, especially if they have been seasick. With water at a premium, washing is likely to be impossible, but a packet of baby wipes or other moist wipes will help clean your skin of salt and reduce the likelihood of salt-water boils. The inclusion of a few feminine sanitation items may also be appreciated.

Personal identification documents

It is always a good idea, even for those who never go to sea, to scan or take photos on your phone of all important personal documents and ensure they are uploaded to Cloud storage, as well as stored on your phone and/or computer. If you are travelling outside home waters, make sure you have a scan or photo of all crew and guest passports, or other relevant ID and a copy uploaded to the Cloud. Include a hard copy of personal documents in the grab bag. Photocopy the documents onto waterproof paper or laminate ordinary paper, the internet can fail, and telephones can get lost.

Prescription glasses

Pack a spare pair of glasses, in a rigid case, for each crewmember who needs them. Even a not quite current prescription is better than nothing. Include some cheap reading glasses for the longsighted; they can also be very useful for magnifying things.

Personal inspiration

This may be a religious book, a collection of poems, something for meditation or whatever else is appropriate to your beliefs or views. It's a bit like the classic BBC radio programme *Desert Island Discs*, which always allows the castaway to take a book of their choice. However, in their case, the Bible, or other religious work, plus the complete works of Shakespeare, are already on the 'island'. The BBC 'castaway' is also allowed an inanimate luxury item, which has no practical value; perhaps you could include something too, though the most popular choice of a piano might be a bit impractical!

Personal medicine

Include a supply of any drugs required by any of the crew in the grab bag, being sure to rotate them regularly. If the required drugs must be kept refrigerated, make sure they are stored in as accessible a position as possible, in a watertight container and add it to the Last-minute Grabs list. It is difficult to know exactly how much to pack, especially as lack of food and water can affect the actions of drugs, perhaps 30 days for an ocean grab bag and five days for a coastal bag.

Spare clothing

Everyone should be wearing as many layers of clothing as possible before taking to the liferaft, but in a very rapid exit some people might not have time to dress warmly. Extra clothes packed in a watertight bag are a bonus, especially if it is necessary to enter the water. A vacuum-bagging machine can reduce a fleece to a very small size and ensures it stays completely dry.

Sunglasses

A pair of sunglasses for each crewmember need not cost a lot, but will be very welcome if it's warm and sunny. One pair for the watchkeeper is vital.

Yacht's papers

As with your personal documents, it is also sensible to store scans of your yacht's registration, insurance documents and any other important paperwork on your phone, computer and in the Cloud. As with Personal Identification Documents, include a copy of the yacht's registration and any other official documents (photocopied onto waterproof paper or on ordinary paper and laminated) in your grab bag. Sharing a set with the holder of your Voyage Details Plan or Designated Person Ashore is also sensible.

▶ Miscellaneous

These items do not fit anywhere else or, like duct tape they overlap several categories.

Batteries

Including spare alkaline batteries for all electrical equipment has been mentioned with individual items, but it is reiterated here as a reminder. Make sure you rotate these batteries regularly with the yacht's supply. Rechargeable batteries can be refreshed using a solar panel charging device.

Camera

If you have a little spare room, pack a waterproof sports camera in your grab bag. If your mobile phone won't take videos or photos for some reason, you'll still be able to record what happened in the liferaft for your social media account!

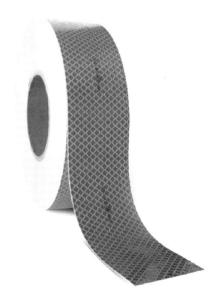

▶ Adhesive tape is often invaluable.

Contents list

As well as marking everything inside your grab bag in waterproof ink you need to include a complete contents list. Detail everything inside your grab bag and print the list on waterproof paper or laminate it.

Include brief instructions on how to use and maintain each item where appropriate. Place the list at the top of the grab bag, and a second copy in the onboard Training Manual. Place a third copy in the Maintenance Record Book with expiry dates of all items. Make a digital pdf and ensure everyone on board downloads a copy to the their portable devices, and also send it to your shoreside contacts. Your Designated Person Ashore (DPA) can share this list with the rescue services in the event of an emergency, so they understand you have the potential to survive a long time.

Do not forget to update the contents list whenever you make any changes to the grab bag.

Duct tape

This is also known as 'elephant tape' and books have been written in honour of its many uses. Get the very best quality tape you can find, two rolls at least, as you will want one for the yacht if you don't already have it aboard. Test that the type you choose will stick in the wet as some brands are better than others. You can use this tape for all sorts of repairs and improvisations such as:

- Liferaft leaks above the waterline.

- Securing a bandage or split to a patient.
- Covering the strobe light on an EPIRB.
- Taping containers to obtain a completely watertight seal.

Foil

A large sheet of thick aluminium foil, folded up, takes up little room and has many uses, including radar reflection and fishing lures.

Plastic bags

It would be difficult to pack too many plastic bags. We acknowledge they are not environmentally friendly, but in your liferaft they will be invaluable. Include a selection from huge to tiny together with plenty of assorted sized, resealable, heavy weight, freezer bags (the zipper style and re-sealable silicone bags are particularly easy to use).

▶ Last-minute Grabs

Some of the things in the other categories may also belong here on your boat, as they, or additional units, are going to be stored outside your grab bag. Your Last-minute Grabs list should be pinned up in a prominent position aboard your yacht. Create a list to ensure you do not forget something essential when you abandon ship. See page 51 for an example of one such list.

Binoculars

You could pack a spare pair in your grab bag, but it is more likely that you will take those from the yacht. They will help you make sure you are seeing a genuine rescue craft before you set off a flare.

Cockpit cushions

These can add to comfort and warmth in the liferaft, especially if it lacks an insulated floor. Buoyant cushions, such as the US Type IV personal flotation device, can also be used to help survivors in the water.

EPIRB

Collect the yacht's EPIRB from its hydrostatic holder or any other EPIRB stored outside the grab bag. The more EPIRBs you have in your liferaft, the better.

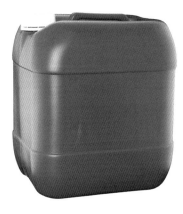

▶ If possible, fill every container with drinking water and leave alcohol behind.

Extra food and drink

Grab as much as you can from the galley, especially the cookie jar and other carbohydrates. Add as many soft drinks and cartons of long life milk as you can, and do not forget any large

SAMPLE 'LAST-MINUTE GRABS' LIST

Equipment	Location
EPIRB	Aft deck in float free holder
Bottled water	Aft deck locker
Buckets	Aft deck locker
Man overboard sling	Aft deck, port side
Horseshoe lifebuoys	Aft, port & starboard side
Down blankets	Cockpit
Cockpit cushions	Cockpit
Flares container	Cockpit
Spear gun	Rack behind cockpit
Portable VHFs (2)	On charge in workshop
Medical kit	Skipper's cabin
Passports & cash	Safe in skipper's cabin
Fleece blankets	Individual cabins
Lifejackets	Individual cabins
Mobile phones & tablets	Individual cabins
Spare warm clothing	Individual cabins
Torches, head	Individual cabins
USB charging cables	Individual cabins
Heavy weather gear	Wet gear locker
Binoculars	Chart table
Radio	Main saloon, starboard aft locker
Extra food & drink	
Cookie jar, fruit, chocolate, breakfast cereals	Galley
Long life milk and soft drinks	Under floor, aft saloon
Tinned food, dried fruit	Starboard seating in main saloon
Any other food to hand	Galley fridge, stores locker
John's prescription drugs	Galley fridge, top shelf

water containers you have stored on deck. If there is time, fill every possible container with drinking water. Leave the alcohol behind; it can wait for the survival celebration once you are safely ashore.

Fleece blankets

Many small yachts use fleece blankets as bedding and these are ideal for extra warmth in a liferaft, even if it they are slightly damp.

Heavy weather gear

Even if you are in the tropics, make sure everyone has put their waterproofs on top of layers of clothing, before leaving the yacht. It can be cold at night. The higher your latitude and colder the water the more you should put on to protect yourself from hypothermia.

Immersion suit

In cold waters (those less than 21°C (70°F)), an immersion or survival suit is highly recommended. Remember that some immersion suits are not insulated, and it is essential that warm clothing be worn before putting on the suit. In theory, survival suits should be in the grab bag, but they are often large and each can usually be considered as a separate stand-alone grab bag.

Lifejacket

Without a lifejacket even an Olympic champion swimmer will have difficulty staying afloat in cold water because of the disabling effects of cold, shock and cramp. A lifejacket:

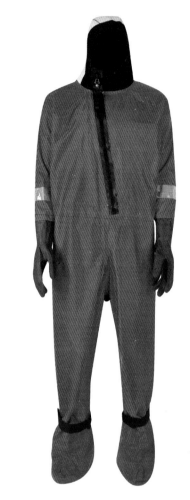

▶ An immersion suit is recommended for water colder than 21°C (70°F).

- Should comply to ISO 12402.
- Will keep you afloat without effort or swimming, regardless of how much clothing you are wearing.
- Must be of sufficient buoyancy for your possible sailing conditions.
- Should be carried for everyone aboard your yacht, including any children.

- Must be worn if abandoning ship is a possibility, in case you end up in the water.
- Can serve as a cushion to sit on inside the liferaft.

Man overboard buoy

This can be used for its original purpose, to attract attention, but also to jury rig a mast or to hold up a radar reflector or SART.

Medical kit

Ideally, this will be in a waterproof and sealed container, which will make it easier to transfer to the liferaft. If the medical kit is packed in something less impermeable to water, consider purchasing a better box before you sail. The sea is a damp environment even aboard a large yacht and medical equipment can be spoiled very quickly. Remember to take the prescription drugs container if that is stored in a different location.

Portable GPS

With celestial navigation fast becoming a dying art, most yachts now carry at least one handheld device with built-in GPS. These include smartphones, portable tablet computers and even smartwatches. Knowing where exactly you are in a liferaft is nice, even if you cannot influence where you are going. Make sure your device is waterproof or kept in a waterproof case.

Portable VHF

A survival craft radio is included in the Search and Rescue category, but even if your grab bag includes one, you should still take any other portable VHFs to the liferaft. The ideal VHF should be:

- Waterproof and buoyant.
- Fitted with GPS, DSC and AIS.
- Fitted with a lithium-ion battery.
- Kept fully charged.
- Capable of using alkaline batteries as well as rechargeable ones.

Radio

Many yachts, especially those engaged in blue water cruising, have a short-wave portable radio on board to listen to commercial stations. Packed in a waterproof bag, this can provide morale boosting entertainment in a liferaft. Don't forget to include the correct spare batteries in the grab bag.

Telephones

While a mobile cellular or portable satellite telephone should not be your only means of making a call for help, they may be valuable additional methods of making contact when you are in a liferaft. Make sure you have a floating waterproof case to protect the phone, and a charged spare battery. Inmarsat and Iridium both have satellite telephones that can be used to make distress calls even though, like cellular telephones, they are not primarily designed to do so.

 Packing a spare charged battery is really important.

Tablet computer

If you have thought ahead you will have downloaded useful information onto your tablet. Take it with you, if only for the maps and survival information you will have downloaded and stored. You never know, there might even be a movie you can watch or a book you can read to while away the time before rescuers sail over the horizon towards you. Do remember that most portable devices such as these are somewhat shy of water.

Spare clothing

If there are no, or very few, spare clothes packed in the grab bag make sure they are on your Last-minute Grabs list.

Spear gun

Those who fish at sea for food and not for fun, often keep a spear gun aboard. While its main function is usually below water, it is an excellent method of killing a large fish caught when trawling, as well as providing an extra line to help bring it aboard. A spear gun used above water must be powered by bands rather than compressed air, which is only suitable for underwater use. If you carry a spear gun, include it in your Last-minute Grabs, as it can be used to catch the fish attracted to your liferaft. Make sure your grab bag is one of the places you store spare bands, shafts and tips.

▶ Shopping Lists

To help you decide how much or how little to include in your grab bag, suggested shopping lists for different voyages and locations are shown on the following pages.

The Ocean Grab Bag

The ultimate bag for round the world cruising and ocean passage making. It includes everything detailed in this chapter.

The Coastal Grab Bag

This assumes all passages are close to shore where rescue will be measured in hours, or at worst a day or so in less populated areas. This grab bag could also be used for short passages further offshore, especially with the addition of some water.

Warm Water Variation

Ideal for those sailing in tropical waters, where the risk of hyperthermia is low.

The Cold Weather Variation

This version is for sailors living in a temperate or colder climate, especially those who sail in the winter season.

The Minimalist Grab Bag

This list is for those with the best liferaft money can buy and the appropriate GMDSS equipment for their sailing area. It assumes you can send an automated distress message using the on-board DSC radio and satellite communications equipment. Wherever you are in the world help should arrive soon, but just in case it is delayed for any reason a watermaker is included. Meanwhile, with your portable satellite phone you can use your time in the raft to sell your survival story to the media!

▶ *Maintenance and Service*

A grab bag is not a 'buy and forget about it' item of safety equipment; like a liferaft it also needs regular maintenance and money outlay to keep it in perfect condition. When your liferaft is away having its annual service, you should unpack your grab bag and check all items, too. Electronic items should be checked even more frequently.

Your EPIRB

To guarantee your EPIRB has every chance of operating correctly if an emergency occurs you should, for each beacon:

- Ensure you and your crew know exactly how it works.
- Register it and update the information as necessary.
- Ensure it is stored or secured so that it cannot be accidentally switched on. This is the main cause of expensive time-wasting false alerts.
- Once a week, visually inspect for signs of damage or corrosion.
- Once a month, and before any long passages, activate the self-test.
- At the start of a season and before any long passage, check the battery and any hydrostatic release. Change them if the expiry date is close.

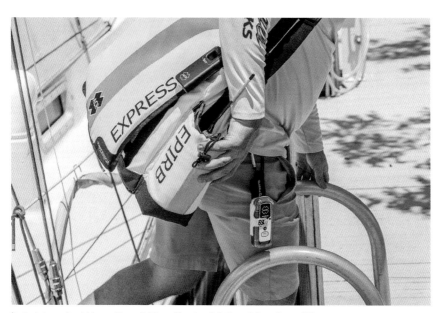

▶ Grab bags should be easily portable and kept as light in weight as is possible.

OCEAN GRAB BAG LIST

Search & Rescue

EPIRB x 2
Flare – LED
Flares – buoyant orange
  smoke x 2
Flares – red handheld x 6
Flares – red parachute x 6
Flashlight + spare
  batteries x 3
Kite – parafoil
PLB

Radar Reflector

Rescue line & quoit
SART
SOLAS signal table
Signalling mirror 1pp
Strobe light
VHF
Whistle x 2

Maintenance & Protection

Bailer x 2
Bucket
Chemical heat pack 2pp
Diving mask x 2
Inflatable cushions
Light sticks x 8
Paddle x 2
Pump x 2
Repair kite
Rope, assorted
Safety knife
Sail repair tape
Sea anchor x 2
Sponges 1pp
Sunscreen
TPA 1pp
Umbrella
Watch hat

Medical

Medical
Anti-seasickness tablets
  6pp+
Enema kit
First aid kit
Petroleum Jelly
Seasickness bags
Sunburn cream

Food & Drink

Can opener x 2
Containers, assorted
Cutlery 1pp
Cutting board
Drinking cup 1pp
Drinking water 1.5l pp
Fishing kit
Food rations
Funnel
Gloves
Multivitamin tablets 30pp
Solar still
Watermaker

Survival & Morale

Battery bank x 2
Charts
Compass
Knife
Knife sharpener
Land survival book
Land survival kit
Lighter
Multipurpose tool
Pack of cards
Pens & pencils x 4
Scissors
Solar chargers x 2
Survival instructions
Towels x 2
Waterproof paper pad x 2

Personal

Contact lens kit
Condoms
Credit card
Money
Personal hygiene supplies
Personal ID
Prescription glasses &
  reading glasses
Personal inspiration
Personal medicine
Spare clothing
Sunglasses
Yacht's papers

Miscellaneous

Batteries
Camera
Contents list
Duct tape
Foil
Plastic bag

Note: Delete from this list
any items already packed
inside your liferaft, if known
to be of excellent quality

COASTAL GRAB BAG LIST

Search & Rescue

EPIRB
Flare – LED
Flare – orange smoke
Flares – red handheld x 3
Flares – red parachute x 3
Flashlight x 2
Kite – parafoil
PLB

Radar Reflector

Rescue line & quoit
SART
Signal card
Signalling mirror x 2
Strobe light
VHF
Whistle x 2

Maintenance & Protection

Bailer
Bucket
Chemical heat pack 1pp
Light sticks x 2
Paddle x 2
Pump
Repair kit
Rope, assorted
Safety knife
Sea anchor x 2
Sponges x 2
Sunscreen
TPA 1pp
Watch hat

Medical

Anti-seasickness tablets
First aid kit
Seasickness bags

Food & Drink

Boiled sweets
Containers, assorted
Drinking cup 1pp
Drinking water 0.5l pp
Energy/fruit bars

Survival & Morale

Battery bank and
  charging cables
Compass
Knife
Knife sharpener
Land survival book
Land survival kit
Lighter
Multipurpose tool
Pens & pencils x 2
Scissors
Solar charger
Survival instructions
Waterproof paper

Personal

Contact lens kit
Credit card
Money
Personal medicine
Prescription glasses
Sunglasses
Yacht's papers

Miscellaneous

Batteries
Camera
Contents list
Duct tape
Plastic bag

Note: Delete from this list
any items already packed
inside your liferaft, if known
to be of excellent quality

CLIMATIC VARIATIONS TO YOUR GRAB BAG
Cold Weather Variation

Add:	Delete:
• Warm hats	(except in polar regions)
• Gloves	• Sunglasses
• Extra chemical heat packs	• Sunscreen
• Extra food	• Sunburn cream
• Additional spare clothes	
• Immersion suits	

CLIMATIC VARIATIONS TO YOUR GRAB BAG
Warm Water Variations

Add:	Delete:
• Sunhats	• Chemical heat packs
• Extra sunscreen	• Inflatable cushions
• Extra sunburn cream	
• Extra water	
• Sunglasses 1pp	

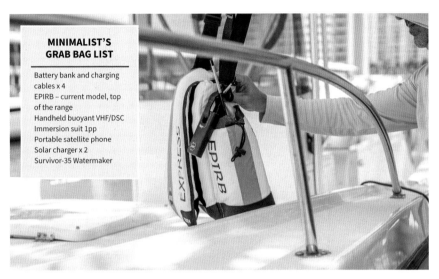

MINIMALIST'S GRAB BAG LIST

Battery bank and charging cables x 4
EPIRB – current model, top of the range
Handheld buoyant VHF/DSC
Immersion suit 1pp
Portable satellite phone
Solar charger x 2
Survivor-35 Watermaker

▶ Always stow the grab bag where it can be easily found in an emergency.

For all safety equipment you should:

- Read any owner's manual.
- File a copy of all instructions and information in the crew training manual.
- Scan and load PDF versions of instruction manuals onto your computer, tablet and/or smartphone.
- Add it to the safety equipment list, which should be displayed in a prominent position.
- Enter the item in your Maintenance Record or Log Book, including where appropriate:
  - An inspections checklist.
  - Maintenance and repair instructions.
  - Maintenance schedule.
  - Lubrication points diagram, plus recommended lubricants.
  - A list of replaceable parts.
  - A list of sources of spare parts.
  - A record of inspection and maintenance.
- Fill in and send off any registration card.
- Mount or stow the item in its correct position immediately.
- If appropriate, practise using the item.

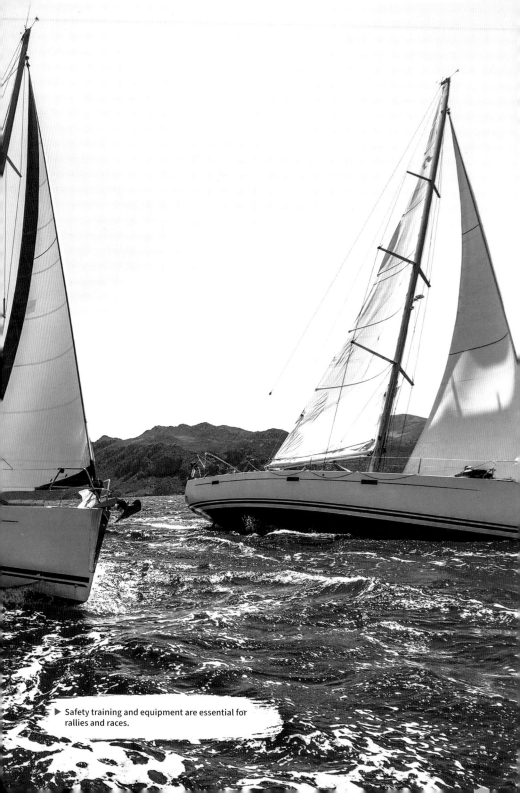

Safety training and equipment are essential for rallies and races.

4 RALLIES AND OCEAN RACES

One of the safest ways to cross an open ocean in a yacht is in the company of other boats, with like-minded people. Bluewater sailing is the dream for most sailors, and more and more specialist companies and organisations are making it easier for anyone to take part in ocean races and rallies.

▶ Rallies

World Cruising Club Rallies

LONG-DISTANCE SAILOR Jimmy Cornell is credited with having created the offshore cruising rally concept in the 1980s and personally organised transatlantic rallies, round the world rallies and even a round the world race.

Over 3,000 boats and 15,000 sailors have participated in sailing events Cornell organised including the Atlantic Rally for Cruisers (ARC), which he first ran under the World Cruising Club (WCC) banner in 1986. Cornell later sold his interests in WCC in 1998, but since that date the ACR has continued to stage regular annual events across the Atlantic, from the Canary Islands to the Caribbean. Typically, 450 boats and 1,500 crew sail with the ARC each year, with some boats and crews proudly proclaiming to have participated on several crossings.

Safety training and equipment

The organisers have strict rules when it comes to what yachts should carry and how crew must be trained.

WCC insist that the skipper, and at least one crewmember, attend courses with both theoretical and practical sessions in emergency communication, pyrotechnics and signalling gear, along with training in liferafts and abandoning ship.

They require every person on board to have an inflatable combined lifejacket-harness with a sprayhood, crotch strap and three-clip safety line, as well as an AIS personal crew overboard beacon for each crewmember.

Each yacht must carry a range of safety equipment based on the World Sailing Offshore Special Regulations and these include:

- A 406 MHz EPIRB.
- Means of sending and receiving email at sea.

- An AIS transponder.
- Man-overboard equipment.
- One or more offshore, self-inflating liferaft with sufficient capacity for at least all the crew on board.

The liferafts must meet one of the following standards:

- ISO 9650 Type 1 Group A with liferaft emergency pack ISO >24 hours, or equivalent, made up of ISO <24 hours and a grab bag.
- ISAF liferafts, manufactured before 2016 until replacement is due at end of service life, plus food and water equivalent to ISO >24 hours.
- SOLAS liferaft with SOLAS 'A' pack.

Each raft must be mounted externally or capable of being at the lifelines ready to launch within 15 seconds. Additionally, for multihulls, the raft must be deployable whether inverted or not. Liferafts are inspected to ensure compliance, correct stowage and in-service, during the pre-departure safety equipment inspection.

Grab bag

When it comes to grab bags, WCC insist that each yacht have one for every liferaft it carries. These bags should have inherent flotation, be marked with the name of the yacht, and have a lanyard and clip attached.

Each grab bag must contain:

- Additional drinking water in a dedicated and sealed container, or a hand-operated desalinator, plus containers for water.
- Additional high energy food.
- Daylight signalling mirror and signalling whistle.
- EPIRB.

- First aid kit, including sunscreen and medical supplies for pre-existing medical conditions.
- Graduated plastic drinking vessel for rationing water.
- Light sticks x 2, or watertight flashlight x 2.
- Polythene bags.
- Red handheld flares, compliant with SOLAS, which may be LED x 2.
- Safety can openers (if food or water is in cans) x 2.
- Sea anchor and line.
- Seasickness tablets.
- String.
- Waterproof handheld VHF transceiver.
- Watertight flashlight with spare batteries (and bulb if not LED).

The Oyster Round the World Rally

Oyster Yachts build bluewater cruising yachts, so it is not surprising that the company should organise a world encircling rally. It enables owners of their yachts to sail safely around the world together with like-minded souls who also own an Oyster yacht. The Oyster Round the World Rally (OWR) is a complete circumnavigation with the reassurance of being part of a large fleet of similar yachts, and the added benefit of service and support from the builder's technical team.

Lasting some sixteen months, the rally's Caribbean start allows yachts to complete the ARC first if so desired. It gets the fleet through the Panama Canal and into the Pacific fairly quickly, maximizing the time visiting the Galapagos Islands and the beautiful Society Islands including Tahiti, Bora Bora and Moorea. From the

Pacific, the fleet head to the Great Barrier Reef, round the top of Australia, Hamilton Island, on to Bali and heading west for Cape Town for Christmas and on to Brazil for carnival before joining up for a final grand party in April.

Safety training and equipment

The organisers specify crew must undertake training in an MCA approved Medical First Aid at Sea course, an SSB/Long Range Radio (GMDSS) course, an RYA Yachtmaster™ Ocean theory course (or equivalent) and a 1-Day Sea Survival course with an in-the-water liferaft drill.

Prior to departure, a series of seminars help participants prepare for the rally. These include key speakers on safety, meteorology, downwind sailing, medical and first aid, insurance, communications and electronics.

The organisers insist that each yacht follows the World Sailing Offshore Special Regulations Category 1 Monohull guidelines when it comes to the carriage of safety equipment, and specifies the carriage of liferafts that meet ISO 9650 standards, and carry a >24-hour pack, with additional grab bag for the above contents. If a yacht has a SOLAS raft, then Oyster recommends that the owner should change it.

Yachts must also be equipped with:
- 406 MHz EPIRB.
- AIS man overboard device (with integrated DSC) fitted to each crewmembers lifejacket.
- AIS Transmitter and receiver.
- Marine VHF fitted radio with emergency antennae.
- Means of receiving and sending emails at sea.
- SSB HF Radio.

- Waterproof handheld VHF/DS Receiver.

Grab bag

OWR insist that if the liferaft onboard has <24-hour emergency pack inside it, then a grab bag is mandatory and must carry the items that are missing from the mandatory >24-hour pack.

The organisers do not insist on yachts carrying a grab bag, believing it to be a matter of individual choice made by each skipper. They do, however, recommend participants pack the following additional items:
- Cash and credit cards.
- Copies of all passports and ship's documents.
- Duct tape.
- EPIRB.
- Extra medical kit items, such as lip salve, sun cream, seasickness tablets, headache pills.
- Handheld GPS and spare batteries.
- Personal medicines.
- Sail repair kit (needles and sail twine).
- Satellite telephone and spare battery (these can be carried from the chart table).
- Spare glasses, for those who need them.
- Sponges.
- Flashlight.
- VHF radio.
- Resealable plastic bags.

▶ *Racing*

Not everyone goes to sea on a transoceanic sightseeing adventure. For some, the oceans are there as a racetrack for a contest where the challenge is to cross it in the fastest possible time. Ocean racing has become a sport embraced by many around the world, and while the household names of Whitbread and Volvo Round the World no longer run as such, others have taken their place and offer the opportunities for thousands of sailors to sign up and cross an ocean in race mode.

Ocean racing is at the mercy of the elements, and these can include extreme weather consisting of high winds and big seas, posing a risk of potential damage to yachts and injury to crew. Good maintenance, operating standards and procedures are used to minimise these risks and ensure that safe working practices are maintained.

The Clipper Round the World Yacht Race

The Clipper Round the World Yacht Race (CRWR) has, since its inception, always placed safety as its number one priority, setting a highly regarded benchmark in the sector by identifying and managing risks. Many crews are attracted by the scale of the challenge and adverse conditions offered by racing across an ocean. Many set out to achieve something remarkable, whether it be a single ocean crossing or an entire circumnavigation. The weather makes no exception for their status; they face the same challenges as any other ocean race and for that reason professional standards are applied throughout. CRWR organisers' aim is to ensure all risks are identified and managed, providing appropriate levels of safety.

Safety training and equipment

Every Clipper Race crewmember will go through exactly the same four levels of training no matter what their previous experience. The training includes an approved Sea Survival course and a classroom-based Advanced Safety Course.

The organisers continually develop and review its standards and procedures so that they meet or exceed those required by the UK's Maritime and Coastguard Agency (MCA). It has also introduced many safety and training initiatives in areas where there are no statutory requirements.

CRWR training is designed to ensure crew can handle the specific demands of large yacht ocean racing so that even novices emerge as very competent sailors. Training also includes an independently provided sea survival course recognised by the RYA and World Sailing.

Clipper Race founder and Chairman Sir Robin Knox-Johnston has stated: 'Sailing can be dangerous, but we train to make it safer, and that's what we do. It's not just in the Clipper Race, it's throughout sailing. We are in fact a very safe activity, but at the end of the day people have to remember those rules, their training and what they've been taught and then it's a safe game. If they start forgetting the rules, then it becomes dangerous.'

Each CRWR yacht carries a maximum of 24 persons on board at any one time, and liferaft capacity is calculated at 150 per cent of the maximum number of people on board.

Grab bag

The location and contents of any grab bags are fully explained as part of the safety brief, which all race crew will receive at every level of their CRWR training, and again when they first join their team and yacht for their respective leg of the race.

As a company, CRWR lays down a list of items that should be carried in a grab bag as standard, and they acknowledge that skippers will add to this list based on their own high-level experience.

Typically, the contents of a Clipper Round the World Race grab bag includes:

- Battery pack for mobile phones.
- Binoculars.
- Cereal bars.
- GMDSS handheld VHF radios.
- Handheld satellite phone plus charger.
- Anti-seasickness tablets.
- Standard handheld VHF radio.
- TPAs.

During predeparture abandon ship drills, all crew are additionally assigned to get certain other items such as required. These items include:

- EPIRB.
- Freshwater containers.
- Medical kit.
- SART.
- Passports (in a dry bag).
- Ship's papers.

The company encourages crew to maintain their own personal items in a dry bag, such as:

- Glasses.
- Medications.
- Mobile phone.
- Wallet.

The Ocean Globe Race

McIntyre Adventure run three around the world yacht races. The Golden Globe Race (GGR), the Ocean Globe Race (OGR) and the Mini Globe Race (MGR). Don McIntyre, the company's founder, is one of Australia's most experienced sailors, having competed in the 1990 BOC Challenge single-handed around the world yacht race, coming second in class, which was the highest placing for an Australian at the time.

Grab bag

For boats racing in the GGR, Don McIntyre recommends a fluorescent orange grab bag with inherent flotation fitted with a lanyard and clip and marked with the yacht's name. The grab bag will contain:

- 12v charge cable.
- Additional 406 MHz EPIRB.
- Additional satellite telephone, handheld with waterproof cover and internal batteries.
- Anti-seasickness tablets, enough for seven days.
- Desalinator, Survivor 06 hand-operated with lanyard and clip.
- First aid kit, clearly marked and resealable.
- Sunscreen.
- Flares – SOLAS, digital or pyrotechnic, in date for at least 12 months:
  - Red handheld flares x 6;
  - White handheld flares x 2;
  - Orange SOLA- compliant smoke flares x 2;
  - Light sticks x 5.
- Food – high energy, minimum 20,000kJ and 20 rehydration electrolyte tablets.

- Medical supplies for pre-existing medical conditions.
- Nylon string, polythene bags.
- SART.
- Safety can opener.
- Sea anchor for the liferaft (not required if the liferaft already has a spare sea anchor in its pack), with four swivel and >30m (98ft) line diameter >7.5mm (0.3in) recommended standard ISO 17339.
- Signalling mirror.
- Glasses, spare unbreakable if needing them.
- Strobe light.
- TPA.
- VHF radio, handheld GMDSS with a long-life battery.
- VHF transceiver, watertight handheld aviation.
- Water containers, 3 x 1l (0.25 gallons) security sealed.
- Wet notebook with captive pencil.
- Whistle.

Portable communication equipment needs to be kept adjacent to the grab bag and be comprised of:

- YB3, a satellite communication device that automatically transmits the yacht's position and sends and receive messages from anywhere with a clear view of the sky.
- Satellite telephone.
- GMDSS VHF.
- Aviation Transceiver.

The Ocean Race

Formerly known as the Whitbread Round the World Race (1973–2001), and then as the Volvo Ocean Race (2001–2019), the Ocean Race have been organising round

the world races every three or four years since 1973. Most recently renamed in 2019, the company organises races with a purpose, and demand the highest possible level of safety requirements. They believe the ocean to be in crisis and have set themselves up to become the catalyst for change by accelerating the protection and restoration of the seas.

Each boat is extensively equipped to cover every possible emergency with the satellite communications, EPIRBs, PLBs, SARTs and handheld VHF radios along with aviation frequency emergency radios.

There is also a long list of other safety equipment that includes liferafts, Jon Buoys for man overboard recovery, extensive medical equipment, flares, a man overboard alerting and positioning system and of course, lifejackets and harnesses.

Contents of the grab bag recommended by the Ocean Race consists of:

- EPIRB.
- SART.
- Flares.
- Radio.
- First aid kit.

▶ Professional Sailors and their Grab Bags

Pip Hare's grab bag

Pip Hare has been a professional sailor since leaving school at 18, and has a career spanning close to 30 years. As well as being a sailor, Pip is a journalist, an author and a motivational speaker. Having sailed the Vendee Globe, she truly understands what is involved when it comes to overcoming challenges to achieve authenticity, risk management and gender equality.

When sailing, Pip carries two EPIRBs, one mounted by the companionway; the other in her grab bag. She carries a PLB on her person and has a personal AIS device fitted to her lifejacket. Her grab bag contains a number of fixed items plus regularly changing extras. She recommends not overloading a bag so there is enough room to find things inside without having to take everything out. Her grab bag includes:

- AIS SART.
- Emergency food rations.
- EPIRB.
- First aid kit.
- Fluorescein dye markers.
- Light sticks.
- GPS personal locator beacon.
- Handheld DSC VHF radio.
- Handheld GPS.
- Red and orange flares.
- Satellite phone with separate SIM card that is reloaded at the start of every trip.
- Second PLB.
- Spare batteries for sat phone and VHF radio in waterproof case.
- Spare batteries in sealed bag.
- Strobe light.
- Survival blankets.
- Flashlight.

Her regularly changed extras in her bag typically include:
- Fishing kit (hooks well protected).
- Lip balms.
- Multitool.

- Narrow diameter string (to hang things up inside the raft).
- Passport.
- Sunscreen.
- Survival blanket for every crewmember.
- Waterproof notepad and pencil.
- Resealable plastic bags.

Pip says, 'It's worth noting that, in the event of abandonment, I'd also aim to put on my immersion suit and lifejacket.'

Nikki Curwen's grab bag

Another offshore racer, Nikki Curwen, has sailed in a Mini Transat solo transatlantic race. As part of class rules, all yachts had to carry a survival container onboard. Inside Nikki's survival container was:

- Fishing equipment.
- Floating smoke signals x 2.
- Handheld VHF (waterproof).
- Knife.
- Light sticks x 3.
- Marine dye marker.
- Parachute flares x 6.
- Red flares x 4.
- Signalling mirror.
- Sunscreen x 2.
- Survival blanket.
- Survival food 500g per person.
- Waterproof torch.

Nikki says, 'We also had to carry a 9l (2.4 gallon) container of survival water, in a 10l (2.6 gallon) canister so it floats. We were potentially days away from help, in the middle of an ocean, so it was quite substantial. And I added anti-seasickness tablets, a GPS and a chocolate bar!'

RNLI

Even the Royal National Lifeboat Institution (RNLI) all-weather lifeboats have grab bags on board. On the boat, there is also a handheld VHF, flashlights and some parachute flares, which crew are trained to take with them in an emergency.

The Shannon-class lifeboat has a big yellow grab bag, containing:

- Handheld flares, for use in day and night x 4.
- Red pinpoint flares, for signalling location x 6.
- Anti-seasickness tablets.
- White flares x 15.

Lifejackets worn by RNLI crew are fitted with a flare and PLB pocket, so these items are always to hand.

Pantaenius Insurance Company

Pantaenius is a specialist yacht insurance provider. Their experts have compiled what they call the definitive grab bag. They believe the grab bag is mainly for personal effects, communication and safety equipment. It includes:

- Bandages.
- Credit card.
- Disinfectant solution.
- Documents, copies of identity and boat papers.
- Food – long-lasting, high-energy items such as nuts, dried fruits, chocolate and energy bars.
- Handheld flares.
- Handheld GPS and compass – do not forget batteries!
- Hat.
- Healing ointment.
- Heat packs.
- Important spare keys.
- Knife, ideally one that folds closed.
- Light – long-range visible sparkling light (40 to 60 flashes per minute).
- Painkillers.
- Pen, waterproof that can be used to write directly on the inner wall of the liferaft.
- Radio – waterproof, handheld, DSC-enabled and equipped with a GPS receiver.
- Rescue blankets – metal-coated, lightweight.
- Ropes.
- Sea sickness remedies.
- Sun protection.
- Sunscreen, high protection factor to protect against sunstroke and sunburn.
- Sunglasses.
- Tape – heavy duty, waterproof.
- Toothpaste and toothbrushes.
- Torch, waterproof.
- Water in canisters about 80 per cent full, attached to and float beside the liferaft.
- Webbing, can be used to secure people or objects to the liferaft.

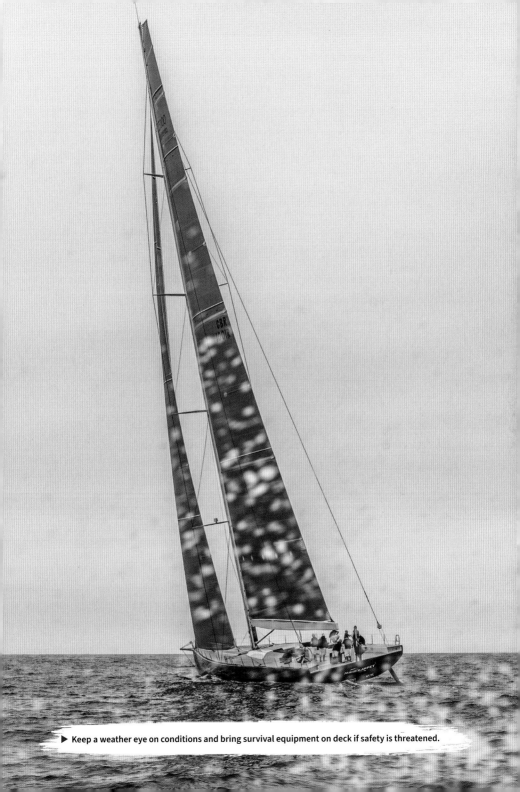

► Keep a weather eye on conditions and bring survival equipment on deck if safety is threatened.

5 ABANDONING SHIP

Collision, fire, flooding and grounding are four of the possible reasons why the skipper of any yacht may have to utter those two words that every sailor dreads: 'Abandon ship'. This chapter discusses what to do from the moment the skipper gives that order to prepare to abandon ship, until such time as everyone is safely on board the liferaft.

WHETHER YOU SAIL alone or with a large crew, you should have at least given some thought as to how to cope with a disaster and, at best, performed regular practise drills of likely scenarios. In an emergency, the human brain falls back on well-learned patterns of behaviour. This is good news for trained crew, but can have unfortunate consequences for untrained people who may react with inappropriate behaviour. On page iii there is an Emergency Flowchart for an abandon ship situation; it can be used for practise and real situations. Remember it is always better to remain with your boat:

- A boat is bigger than any liferaft she carries.
- It can better withstand the sea and provide shelter for people.
- It is more easily detectable by the SAR units.
- Crew taking to a liferaft have been lost, whilst the deserted vessel remained afloat.

In some situations, for example an out-of-control fire, it may be prudent to take to the liferafts and may later be possible to return to the mother ship.

▶ Emergency Signals

It is vitally important that in an emergency you can quickly gather all the crew together. Even on a small boat, someone shouting from the wheel when the engine is running is unlikely to be heard by any crew below. It is important to consider an alternative method of summoning everyone, for example a handheld foghorn or whistle.

An urgent situation

When an emergency arises, the skipper must take charge. Ideally, the skipper will be in control and organising matters rather than actually doing the work. With a small crew the skipper will not have that luxury, but they must:

- Delegate as much as possible.
- Keep an overall picture of the situation.
- Be ready to take immediate action to maintain the safety of life.

> The skipper should always be guided by their primary responsibilities:
> - The safety of those entrusted to their care.
> - The safety of the boat.
> - The protection of the marine environment.
>
> All other considerations are secondary to these.

Trying to cure the problem must take a very high priority, but an early and immediate attempt should be made to contact other people, such as rescue services and nearby vessels, to alert them to the situation and request assistance. A vessel or crew with a serious problem, but not yet in a distress situation, should send a Pan Pan message rather than a Mayday.

Vessels with DSC can initiate a Pan Pan following the procedure outlined in the appropriate equipment manual. On a DSC VHF this is done as follows:

- Press MENU
- Scroll to ALL SHIPS CALL (to broadcast to all DSC enabled stations and vessels in range)
- Press ENTER
- Scroll to URGENCY
- Press ENTER
- Press ENTER again to confirm (the message has been sent)

The digital message sent will include your MMSI number but **NOT** your position. DSC equipment will repeat the message every four minutes until a digital acknowledgement is received or the alert is cancelled.

After sending the DSC alert, wait 15 seconds and then give a voice Pan Pan call and message over the radio including the position of the vessel. This will ensure everyone in receipt of the alert will know the location of the vessel, and anyone nearby without DSC will also receive the alert.

▶ *Preparing to Abandon Ship*

If it is clear that the accident or emergency situation is not going to be resolved, or that there is even a slight possibility that

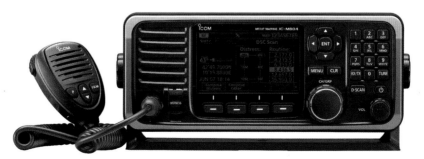

▶ An IC-M804 controller.

the situation may escalate and become out of control, the skipper must prepare to abandon ship. In the best of all worlds, with a large crew, the various jobs can be carried out while a part of the crew continues to try to save the vessel. With a small crew it may be necessary to cease attempting to cure the problem and get on with preparing to leave the vessel.

Avoiding hypothermia and drowning

The two major threats for people abandoning ship are hypothermia and drowning. COLD, not lack of food and water, is the greatest killer after abandoning ship. People become too cold to help themselves in the water, and drown. After boarding a survival craft, even if crew never entered the water and became wet, they can still die of cold if the necessary precautions have not been taken. The epic survival voyages, which have attracted publicity in the past, have nearly all taken place in tropical waters.

If it should be necessary to enter the water on abandoning the vessel, the initial 'cold shock' may prove disabling or even fatal. Extra clothing will prolong your survival time by reducing loss of body heat. Everyone must:

- Put on extra layers of clothing, ideally:
  - a lightweight base layer of wool or synthetic fibre that wicks away moisture;
  - a thicker mid-layer, again made of wicking fibres such as wool or fleece;
  - avoid cotton that loses all insulating properties once wet.

- Put on foul weather gear, fastening tightly at the wrist and ankles (with duct tape if necessary).
- Add socks, shoes, gloves, hat etc.
- Best of all, wear an immersion suit.
- Finally, add your lifejacket.

Lots of clothes will not weigh you down – in fact the opposite is true. When you enter the water, the air trapped between the extra layers of clothing will help your lifejacket keep you afloat. Even if you board the survival craft without getting wet, the extra clothing will help to save your life while awaiting rescue. If possible, pack spare clothes in a dry bag in case you have to swim; this bag can also be used as a substitute flotation device.

Survival in cold water is time limited and there is a clear correlation between water temperature, thermal protection, high body mass and partial immersion. For normally clothed individuals, the following survival times are generally used by search and rescue organisations. At the lower figure, 50 per cent are expected to survive, and the higher is approaching 0 per cent:

Water Temperature	Survival Time
5°C (41°F)	1–6 hours
15°C (59°F)	6–18 hours
20–30°C (68–86°F)	over 24 hours

Preparing the liferaft

There are too many stories of crews launching a liferaft and tying it alongside to await orders, only to have it swept away before anyone boarded. During the disastrous 1998 Sydney—Hobart Race, the yacht *Naiad* inflated her two liferafts and tethered them to the yacht on the leeward side. A large wave struck the *Naiad*, and the liferafts quickly vanished. Liferafts have pockets on the bottom that are designed to fill quickly with water and restrain the liferaft from moving freely through the water. When tied to a moving yacht, the liferaft will naturally resist being pulled through the water. Immense strain is placed upon the tether or its anchor point, one of these will eventually fail.

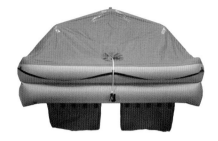

▶ An inflated ocean ISO 8-man liferaft (back).

The liferaft must not be launched until such time as the abandon ship order is given by the skipper, but it must be made ready. Depending upon where a liferaft is stowed normally:

- Release the securing arrangements.
- Move the raft to the launch position:
  - The lowest deck.
  - Amidships on the leeward side.
  - The stern in a calm sea if the boat has a swimming platform.
- Do not inflate the raft on deck:
  - The exploding canister can cause injuries.
  - The raft could get jammed.
  - Parts of the yacht could pierce the raft.
- Make the painter fast to a strong point, such as a mooring cleat, but definitely not to the lifelines, which could easily break under a strain.

If time permits launch any dinghies, surfboards, canoes or anything else that floats and tie them alongside, ready to use or later attach to the liferaft.

Assembling the survival kit

This is where the Last-minute Grabs list (see page 51) is invaluable as a memory

aide. Use it while collecting various articles such as binoculars, EPIRB, food and water, medical kit, portable VHF, mobile devices etc. Make sure every item that can has a long lanyard attached to it. Try to collect everything together with the grab bag, ready to transfer to the liferaft.

If time permits, delegate one person to hand out anti-seasickness tablets with water or a soft drink. A liferaft can affect even the strongest stomach, and most medicine is only effective before seasickness sets in. Encourage everyone to drink as much water as possible before leaving the yacht, as this will increase the level of body fluids and will also help overcome the possibility of urine retention due to 'mental blockage' later when in the very public confines of a crowded raft.

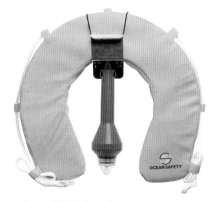

▶ An LBU0120 horseshoe.

▶ *Summoning Help*

Once it becomes obvious that the yacht cannot be saved, assistance must be summoned. If a Pan Pan message was sent it is time to upgrade it to a Mayday.

A DSC VHF is the best choice to make the initial distress alert, and this is usually done by pressing the DSC distress button. With a few extra seconds of time the alert can be 'designated', meaning the nature of the distress can be included eg, collision, fire, sinking etc. It will broadcast a piercing alarm and the yacht's position to other vessels and the authorities.

After sending a DSC distress, the radio will wait for an acknowledgement on channel 70 and receive calls on channel 16. The distress message will be automatically repeated every four minutes, until it is acknowledged.

A DSC distress alert should be followed by a Mayday voice message on channel 16 to give further details and alert any non-DSC equipped vessels nearby. If the vessel does not have DSC, issue a Mayday immediately on VHF (and MF or HF if available).

Use the internationally recognised Mayday format as it ensures all the important information is transmitted; the recipients understand what they hear even if English is their second language.

If the main VHF loses electrical power, or the yacht is dismasted, try using a handheld VHF which ideally will have DSC, though due to the aerial size it will not transmit as far.

When contact has been made by radio or satellite do not cause confusion by also activating your EPIRB unless:

- Contact is lost.
- You are told to do so by the rescue authority.
- The radio ceases to work due to total electrical failure, demasting etc.

If no direct voice contact can be made for whatever reason:

- Set off the vessel's EPIRB.
- Use any of the recognised Distress Signals (see page 136) to attract attention.
- If no vessel is in sight, consider firing two parachute flares:
  - The first flare to catch someone's eye.
  - The second, three minutes later, to give them a direction.
  - Do not waste any more until you know help is nearby.

Using a mobile phone

If it is impossible to make voice contact via radio and the yacht is close to the shore, try making an emergency call by mobile phone.

Even if the mobile phone shows no service, an emergency number automatically uses any available network

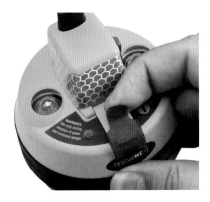

▶ Breaking the tab on an EPIRB1.

and is given priority, so the call may still be able to connect. In certain countries or regions, your location information (if determinable) may be accessed by emergency service providers when you make an emergency call. All phones can be used to make an emergency call, even if locked.

On iPhone 8 or later:
- Press and hold the side button and one of the volume buttons until the Emergency SOS slider comes up.
- Drag the Emergency SOS slider to call emergency services. If you continue to hold down the side button and volume button, instead of dragging the slider, a countdown begins and an alert sounds.
- Hold the buttons until the end of the countdown and the iPhone will automatically call emergency services.

On an earlier model iPhone, or Android:
- On the Passcode screen tap 'Emergency' ('Emergency Call' on Android).
- Dial 999 or 112.
- Ask for the Coastguard.

If the yacht or one of the people aboard has a satellite phone it can be used to make a call to the emergency services.

▶ Staying with the Yacht

While this book is about abandoning ship, it does not mean you should always take to your liferaft. Your liferaft is the final ultimate retreat; it is NOT the first choice when things go wrong. **Never abandon ship until the last possible moment**.

Remember:
- Your yacht is bigger and safer than your liferaft.
- Help may arrive to fight a fire or bring a pump to deal with flooding.
- You may be able to transfer to another vessel or helicopter without ever inflating your raft or getting your feet wet.

▶ Abandoning the Yacht

The skipper is the only person who should give the abandon ship order. No matter how large the boat, this command must only be issued by word of mouth to prevent any possibility of confusion.

Once the abandon ship order is given, but before the liferaft is actually launched, the skipper should:
- Ensure the engine(s) and propeller(s) are stopped.
- Take a note of the position of the yacht to take to the liferaft.
- Make a final Mayday call to announce the abandonment.
- Check everyone aboard is gathered and dressed in warm clothes or immersion suits.
- Check lifejackets are correctly fitted and tightly secured.

Yachts have been reboarded after being abandoned following fire etc. Therefore, time permitting and where appropriate:
- Shut all watertight compartments.
- Close all fuel valves.

Launching the liferaft

Once the order is given to abandon ship, the liferaft must be launched. If possible, get two or three people involved as a liferaft is heavy and awkward, especially in rough seas. Where the liferaft needs to be moved to the launching position choose the windward aft quarter.

To manually launch a liferaft:
1 Check, then double check, the painter is secured to a strong point.
2 Check all fastenings are undone, including the hydrostatic release unit if fitted.
3 Check the water in the launching area is clear of people or obstructions.
4 Throw the raft over the side.
5 Pull the painter until it feels stuck, then pull harder to fire the CO2 bottle and inflate the liferaft. If the liferaft inflates inverted, take the action given on page 78 to right it.
6 If possible, use the painter to pull the raft alongside. This may be difficult in rough weather.
7 Protect the raft from chafing on the side of the yacht and damaging the fabric.

Boarding the liferaft from the yacht

Unloaded liferafts tip over easily, especially before the ballast bags are full of seawater. It is important to get someone heavy aboard as soon as the raft is fully inflated and before any excess gas starts to vent from the overflow valves. Boarding the liferaft without entering the water is the priority to avoid hypothermia or drowning.

Once the first person is aboard the raft, the order in which you transfer everyone else, plus the grab bag, Last-minute Grabs etc, will depend on circumstances and crew numbers.

Actions to take:
• Check no one has any sharp objects that could damage the liferaft.
• Leave injured survivors until last – other crew may land on them and make the injuries worse.
• Climb aboard using a ladder or rope if stepping down is impossible. Do not jump onto the liferaft – this could harm you, the raft canopy or other people already inside.
• Tie lanyards, attached to all equipment, to the yacht or liferaft before passing the item from boat to raft.
• Tie water containers (80 per cent full) onto the outside of the raft to float.
• Attach dinghies, canoes or other floating water toys to the raft.

Entering the water from the yacht

If there is no time, or for some other reason it is impossible to bring the liferaft alongside the yacht, you must enter the water. Even in the event of a rapid sinking, you must try to find time to put on a lifejacket and warm clothing or an immersion suit.

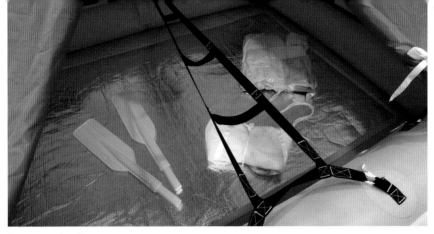

▶ Ocean ISO interior.

When choosing how to leave the yacht, bear in mind:

- Drift of the yacht – if conditions allow, leave on the windward side. A yacht stopped and drifting will make more leeway than you, and swimmers could become trapped by the leeward drift of the vessel.
- Position of any survival craft in the water – remember that the survival craft may drift much more quickly than you can swim.
- Without a survival craft in the water – the stern or bow may be the best choice to get clear of the yacht with more certainty.
- The sea state.
- Other hazards, eg burning oil.

Entering water from a height

Do not jump into the water unless it is essential as sudden immersion into cold water can kill or incapacitate. Use something, such as a ladder, a rope or even a hose, to lower yourself. Slowly entering the water makes the temperature change more gradual.

▶ Action Once in the Water

If you do have to jump:

- Never jump from more than 6m (20ft) wearing an inflated or permanent buoyancy lifejacket.
- Keep your lifejacket on and securely fastened.
- Use one hand to hold down the lifejacket, to stop it hitting your chin on entering the water.
- Always use your other hand to block off your nose and mouth to keep out the water.
- Keep feet together with legs slightly bent.
- Check below to avoid obstructions.
- Jump feet first, looking straight ahead, looking down can make you tumble forward.

Never remain in the water longer than necessary. Get clear of the boat and into a liferaft as quickly as possible.

Remember that:
- Body heat is lost 20 times faster in water than on land.
- Suction from the yacht sinking is a danger.
- There could be an underwater explosion, so get onto any wreckage if you can, or swim on your back.

Never swim aimlessly since exercise increases heat loss as the blood supply to the muscles is increased, and warmed water trapped by any clothing is forced out. Float using the HELP (Heat Escape Lessening Posture) position to minimise heat loss:
- Cross your arms and grip the neck of your lifejacket.
- Cross your ankles and draw your knees up to your chest.
- Keep as much of your body out of the water as possible.

In rough seas float with your back to the wind and sea to reduce wave splashes. Use the whistle and light attached to the lifejacket to attract others. Use the towing loop on the back of the lifejacket to move an injured person. Unite with other survivors and huddle to increase your visibility and warmth:
- Form a circle facing inwards.
- Loop arms through each other's lifejackets.
- Intertwine legs to reduce heat loss.

You could use the **crocodile** position, joining in a straight line to:
- Face the same direction.
- Maintain contact when swimming towards a liferaft for example.

If you are not wearing a lifejacket, float on your back to save energy, grab anything that might help you float and look out for items that may resurface.

Air trapped in your clothing will provide considerable flotation. Retain boots and shoes, if possible, for future protection.

In cold water:
- **Do not** remove any clothes.
- **Do** keep your head out of the water to reduce heat loss.

In warmer water, clothing can be removed and used to make a temporary float. For example:
- Tie knots in the legs of trousers.
- Swing them through the air by the waistband to trap the air.
- Repeat as air is lost.

Oil fire on the water

If you are in oil-covered water that is free of fire, hold your head high to keep oil out of your eyes.

If the oil is burning:
- Paddle or swim against the wind.
- Discard your lifejacket and swim under the water as far as you can.
- When resurfacing to breathe, make a sweeping movement with your hands to force your body clear and cover your eyes, nose and mouth.
- Sweep the flames clear with broad arm movements across the surface, take a deep breath and get underwater again rapidly.
- Swim clear of the area.

Sharks

Fortunately, very few species of shark attack humans without provocation. It is believed that they are very curious and attracted by unusual noise. The highest risk of a shark encounter is when the yacht sinks.

If sharks are in the water with you:
- Get out of the water into the liferaft or onto anything else floating.
- Retain all clothing, especially on the legs and feet, as feet and unclothed areas are attacked first.
- Keep still: move only to keep the shark in sight.
- If swimming is necessary, move with rhythmic strokes.
- In a group, form a circle facing outwards.
- Bind bleeding wounds.
- Avoid urinating. If essential, void small amounts at long intervals.
- Throw vomit as far away as possible, the same with defecation.
- Get into an oil patch.
- If attack is imminent, splash and yell but conserve your strength to fight.
- If attacked, kick and strike the shark, going for the gills and eyes.

Boarding a liferaft from the water

Once you reach the liferaft:
- Put your arm through the grablines – hands quickly numb in cold conditions.
- Use any foot and handholds to help you enter the raft.
- If wearing a lifejacket, submerge yourself to help 'bob up' higher.
- Assist any weak or injured into the liferaft:
  1 Turn the survivor so that their back is against the liferaft.
  2 Those in the liferaft should then grip them under the arms and on top of the shoulders.
  3 'Dunk' the person several times before lifting them in.
  4 People in the water can help keep the survivor upright and push up to help lift them aboard.

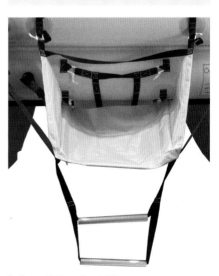

▶ Ocean ISO boarding ladder.

▶ *Righting a Capsized Raft*

A liferaft may inflate in the inverted position, or be capsized by the winds and waves especially if it is empty. Try to right a capsized raft without entering the water, but beware of any potential hazards that could harm the raft. If necessary, move the liferaft into clear water before attempting to right it. One person can easily right a capsized liferaft, even a very large one, from the water in cold conditions.

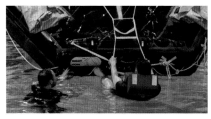

▶ It is possible for one person to right a liferaft.

To right a liferaft:

- Position the raft with the gas bottle at the downwind side.
- Climb onto the raft from a position close to the gas bottle.
- Standing on the gas bottle, grip the righting strap firmly, then stand upright.
- Check the raft is tilted into the wind.
- Lean back and use your body weight to pull the liferaft over.
- As the liferaft falls backwards exit on your back in a right-hand direction
- If the raft comes over on top of you, do not worry. Simply backstroke out from underneath.

WARNING: Do not attempt to clear the underside of the liferaft by a forward movement. This will bring you up against the gas bottle and the buoyancy of your lifejacket could trap you. Beware of the stability pockets, they may contain lead weights.

A fully manned liferaft is unlikely to capsize, provided that the drogue is streamed at an early stage and that the occupants sit with their backs against the sides of the liferaft. If capsize does occur, carry out the capsize drill as above. Do not panic.

The raft will float high in the water and air will be trapped inside. Evacuate the liferaft in an orderly manner.

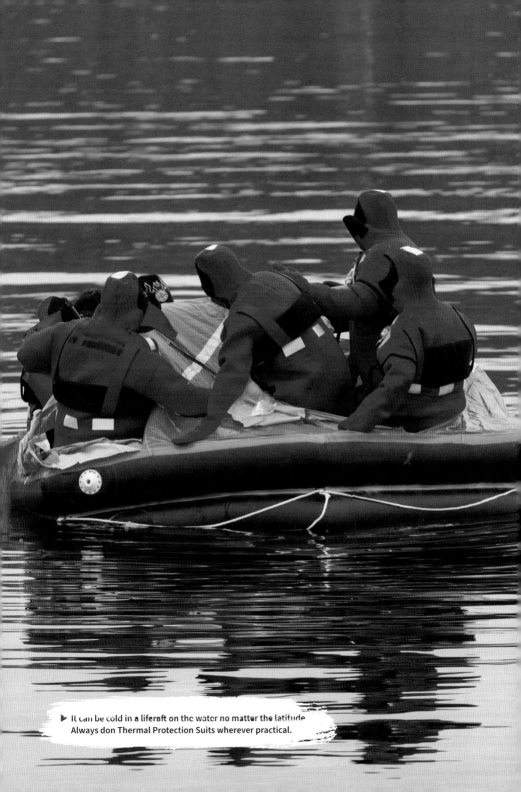

▶ It can be cold in a liferaft on the water no matter the latitude. Always don Thermal Protection Suits wherever practical.

6 INITIAL AND SUBSEQUENT ACTIONS IN THE LIFERAFT

SIMPLY BOARDING A liferaft, especially in rough seas and cold weather, is no guarantee that you will survive. To ensure everyone in a liferaft has some basic information on what to do next, official guidance notes for survival instructions have been included in SOLAS standard liferafts. This chapter expands on these guidance notes with the official wording printed in **_bold italic_**. The information detailing immediate action in a liferaft is given below. A copy should be made and included:

- At the top of every grab bag, laminated or on waterproof paper.
- In any onboard training manual.

The value of training cannot be over emphasised; it will make a real abandon ship situation much less traumatic and give everyone a much better chance of a successful outcome.

> SOLAS instructions for Immediate Action in a liferaft:
> 1 **CUT** the painter and get clear of ship.
> 2 **LOOK** for and pick up other survivors.
> 3 Ensure sea anchor **STREAMED** when clear of ship.
> 4 **CLOSE** the raft entrance.
> 5 **READ** survival instructions.

▶ _Immediate Actions in a Liferaft_

Certain vital actions must be taken as soon as possible after boarding the liferaft:

CUT the painter and get clear of ship

You are in the liferaft because your boat is sinking or burning out of control. You do not want your new home to be hurt by your old one. You must sever your last tie to the mother ship. A safety knife is stowed near each liferaft entrance to cut the painter.

- Cut the painter as far from the raft as possible, the rope may be useful later.
- Pull in the sea anchor if it streamed automatically when the raft inflated.
- Manoeuvre away using the oars or paddles.
- Use the sea anchor to move the raft by throwing the sea anchor in the direction you want to go, and heaving on the hawser to pull the raft towards the sea anchor.

LOOK for and pick up other survivors

Once the raft is clear of the sides of the yacht, check for any more survivors in the water. Establish who, if anyone, is missing. Look for lifejacket lights, listen for whistles or shouts.

With conscious swimmers use the rescue quoit:

- Hold or tie the end of the line in the raft.
- Throw the quoit with its buoyant line to the person in the water.
- Instruct the survivor to put their arm through the quoit, if possible.
- Pull the survivor to the raft.

With an unconscious survivor, or someone unable to hold the quoit, it may be necessary to put someone in the water to help. Do not enter the water without a lifejacket. Take the quoit, leaving the end tied to the raft or held by those aboard. Never underestimate the strength of a panic-stricken person in the water, so always approach a survivor from behind. Use the loop on the back of lifejacket to tow the survivor. Instruct those in the liferaft to pull in both yourself and the survivor. Lift exhausted survivors aboard in the horizontal position, to reduce the chance of a sudden drop in blood pressure.

Ensure sea anchor STREAMED when clear of ship

Stream the sea anchor or drogue as soon as possible to:

- Stabilise the raft.
- Reduce the drift away from survivors who may still be in the water.
- Remain near the last position of the yacht, the likely area of maximum search.
- Reduce the risk of capsize.

Adjust the sea anchor so that when the raft is on a wave crest, the drogue is in the wave trough.

CLOSE the raft entrance

In cold weather, the body heat of occupants will rapidly warm the interior so close entrances when any inflation relief valve has stopped venting. Tie doorway tapes using slipknots to facilitate untying in a hurry.

In tropical climates, leave entrances open to reduce fluid loss caused by perspiration.

READ survival instructions

Everyone aboard the liferaft should, as soon as possible, read all instructions, including this book.

▶ Secondary Actions in a Liferaft

Once the Immediate Actions have been completed, the following secondary actions should be taken as soon as possible. The order in which they are listed here is not necessarily the order in which they should be done; this will depend on the particular circumstances of the situation at the time.

Identify person in charge of liferaft

The skipper from the yacht should be in charge in the liferaft. If that person is missing or disabled, either physically or physiologically, a new leader will have to be selected as soon as possible. Choose someone with a strong will to survive for the good of everyone aboard, and assist them by obeying their orders at once. During the first few hours in the liferaft, survivors will begin to realise what has happened and the danger, injury and possible death that now surrounds them. The skipper must:

- Provide leadership and assurance.
- Prove that they know what to do and have things under control.
- Prevent confusion and social fragmentation.
- Resist depression and sense of failure caused by the loss of the yacht.

Post a lookout

It is essential to post a lookout as soon as possible. They must:

- Look for any missing survivors in the water.
- Watch for other survival craft, SAR vessels, ships or aircraft.
- Scan the water for useful debris.

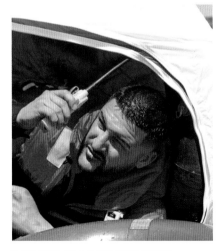

▶ The lookout is watchful for all dangers.

Open equipment pack

Carefully open the liferaft equipment; every item in your liferaft is valuable and irreplaceable. Check the grab bag and whatever else everyone managed to bring before you abandoned ship. If you have an extensive survival kit, look just far enough to find the search and rescue items and anything else you need immediately, consulting the list in your grab bag. A full inventory can wait.

Issue anti-seasickness medicine and seasickness bags

If there was no time to take anti-seasickness tablets while on the yacht, take some immediately. Keep taking these pills for the first 48 hours to avoid any risk of sea sickness and the resultant loss of body fluid. The pills often cause a dry mouth; unless water supplies are plentiful do not issue anything to drink. Anyone affected by seasickness should:

- Put their head down between their knees.
- Try to keep warm.
- Use disposable bags, reducing the smell of vomit that often causes others to be sick.

Dry liferaft floor and inflate, if appropriate

Inevitably, a liferaft will be wet and in rough conditions it is likely to continue getting wet. Bail out as much water as possible and sponge out the rest, reserving at least one sponge if possible. Keep this sponge separate to mop up any condensation as it forms, because this can supplement the water supplies.

In cold conditions, inflate the floor of the raft with the hand pump. If your raft does not have an insulated floor, try to find something to sit on, such as the cockpit cushions.

Administer first aid, if appropriate

Check the physical condition of everyone aboard and give first aid where necessary, remembering the ABCs:

A is for Airway: Is it clear?

B is for Breathing: Are they?

C for Circulation: Is the heart beating? Is there bleeding?

For more information, refer to the first aid notes in Chapter 8.

Manoeuvre towards other liferafts

If there are other liferafts it is important to link them together. Two or more liferafts are much easier for searchers to locate, so connect rafts together with lines. Attached to strong points, eg the painter attachment patch. Allow 15m (50ft) length, or as necessary, to ensure rafts are on wave crests together.

Distribute survivors between the rafts and share out equipment.

Arrange watches and duties

The **skipper** should:

- Establish who is available for watches, note any injuries and the expertise available on board.
- Arrange watches in pairs for about one hour, with an outside lookout and an inside watch if numbers and weather conditions permit.

- Ensure that everyone knows how to keep a lookout and how and when to use all the signalling equipment.
- See that everyone has something to do and is involved when not resting, even if it is only to bail and keep the raft dry.
- Take charge of water and food.
- If possible, record the circumstances leading up to abandoning the yacht.
- Keep a log of events thereafter with times, duties organised, rations issued, first aid given and condition of survivors.

The **lookout** should be:

- Suitably dressed and protected from the elements, with a hat to give shade or warmth, sunscreen applied and sunglasses or a swim mask in rough conditions.
- Well secured to the craft by their harness or a rope.
- Responsible for keeping a lookout for survivors, ships, aircraft and land.
- Watchful for all dangers.
- Collecting any useful debris.
- Alerting everyone to the possibility of rain to collect for drinking.
- Checking for abrasion of liferaft and any attached lines.

The **inside watch** should:

- Look after anyone with injuries.
- Be in charge of the safety and security of all the survival equipment.
- Ensure the signal equipment, particularly the flares, are ready to hand.
- Take responsibility for raft maintenance including bailing, ventilation and repairs.
- Organise the collection of rainwater.

- Supervise the liferaft management while the skipper rests.

Check liferaft for correct operation and any damage

Liferafts are constructed to withstand exposure for 30 days afloat in all sea conditions without deterioration, but they are vulnerable to accidental damage.

- Remove anything sharp or rough from clothing.
- Check frequently for damage from friction of the soles of shoes.
- Take great care when using anything sharp, especially in rough seas.
- Keep all gear stowed properly.
- A well-trimmed liferaft will reduce wear, so spread out evenly around the raft. Sit on the floor with backs to tubes, never sit on the tubes. Use handholds provided as necessary.
- Check regularly for abrasion from anything attached outside – sea anchor, containers of water, other rafts etc.

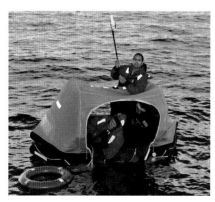

▶ Everybody aboard the liferaft must be ready for the possible arrival of SAR units or the sighting of land.

- Plug and repair holes as soon as possible, following instructions provided with the repair kit in the liferaft emergency pack. Plug large holes, securing them with a hose clamp or string. Use a liferaft repair clamp if available for a quick, permanent repair.
- If a tube has been holed, ventilate the liferaft interior to remove any leaked carbon dioxide.

Check functioning of canopy light and conserve power during daylight

A light on the top of the raft is a valuable aid to location at night. Check that it is functioning and switch it off during daylight hours as it only has a life of between 12 and 24 hours. If your liferaft has no light, or the fitted one has failed, hopefully you will be able to attach the strobe light packed in your grab bag to the top of the raft.

Adjust canopy openings to give protection from weather or to ventilate the liferaft as appropriate

The sea anchor attachment aligns the entrances out of the wind and spray. In warm conditions change the position of the sea anchor line so the raft lies into the wind and open all accesses to give maximum ventilation. Even in cold weather some ventilation will be necessary to provide everyone with plenty of oxygen.

Prepare and use detection equipment including radio equipment

Ensure all signalling equipment is secured at hand, ready for immediate use. The various methods of attracting attention are discussed here; for how to use them once help is close at hand, see Chapter 10.

EPIRB

If your EPIRB is not already on, switch it on now.

- Do not switch the beacon off until instructed by SAR authorities.
- Do not turn the unit off and on to preserve the batteries; it will confuse the rescue authorities and make the final homing very difficult.
- EPIRBs are designed to float outside the raft, attached by a thin line. Ensure the knot is very secure, and check frequently for wear on the line and the raft. In rough weather consider bringing the unit inside the raft.
- If the beacon is kept inside the raft, ensure the liferaft does not have metal foil or metallic lining, which could interfere with the signal. You should:
  - Hold or attach the unit with the antenna vertical.
  - Cover the strobe light to prevent driving the raft occupants crazy.

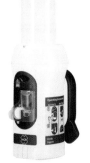

▶ A SART beacon.

- Consider putting the unit outside at night, as the strobe is very effective at guiding rescuers.

SART

Turn the beacon on immediately, it will operate for 96 hours in stand-by mode and in excess of eight hours in operational mode. This should be sufficient time for someone to reach you, except in very remote areas. Attach it as high as possible using:

- Its own pole.
- The man overboard marker buoy from the yacht.
- Anything else available.

Listen for the unit's alarm when it is interrogated by a nearby radar. This is a great morale booster and will alert you to the likelihood of rescuers arriving. It will also give you time to prepare other methods of signalling your whereabouts.

Radar reflector

If you are carrying a radar reflector this should be deployed like a SART, as high as possible in such a position to best reflect the radar signal generated by rescue craft. However, SARTs and radar reflectors conflict with each other and both should not be deployed at the same time.

Portable VHF radio

Conserving your VHF batteries is the priority:

- Send a Mayday as soon as possible, especially if you had previously contacted potential rescuers.
- Keep sending distress signals at regular intervals,

even if you do not receive
a reply.

- If the battery is getting low,
reserve the VHF until help
is close by.
- With a plentiful supply of
batteries, keep the unit on
constantly and send
frequent Maydays.

Pyrotechnics

Flares should not be used unless it is
certain that help is nearby and then,
only when a ship is as close to you as you
think it is likely to get, or, in the case of
an aircraft in daytime, when it is actually
sighted. Take great care, pyrotechnics are
dangerous; they can easy hole a liferaft,
give you a nasty burn and have even killed
people.

Signalling light

Like a pyrotechnic this is best used once
help is close by, as it must be aimed
in the direction of the rescuers to be
effective. A strobe light attached to the
liferaft will be useful for all round vision,
and has the benefit of not needing
any supervision, but its range is more
limited.

Signalling mirror

A signal mirror is inexhaustible and can
be seen for miles; the record rescue
from a mirror is just over 100 miles
(161km). During the daytime the lookout
can catch the sunlight on the mirror
and reflect it around the horizon; with
practise, 270° can be covered with one
mirror. Do not try to use the mirror for
Morse code, as the liferaft is unlikely
to be stable enough. Three flashes in
quick succession are the international
distress signal with a mirror that any
rescuer should recognise.

Kite

If your grab bag includes a parafoil rescue
kite, fly it during the daytime. Tie on the
radar reflector, if the wind is suitable,
as the higher you can suspend this the
better. It may be possible to use the kite
at night to lift a strobe light.

Portable telephones

If you do have a cellular or satellite mobile
phone of any kind, try to call the rescue
services.

Gather up any useful floating objects

All useful debris should be collected;
anything may have value later as an
aid to survival. The most important
items are those that can be used for
signalling, such as EPIRBs or SARTs.
Heavy articles with sharp edges should
not be taken aboard as they could
damage the raft.

Protect against heat, cold and wet conditions

Heat

It is essential in hot weather to keep as
cool as possible to reduce perspiration
and minimise dehydration. Use the
cooling effect of the sea as follows:

- Do not inflate the floor of the raft.
- Regularly wet the liferaft canopy.
- Wet clothes with seawater, but
bear in mind damp clothes increase
susceptibility to skin sores or
saltwater boils.
- Ensure clothes are dry by dusk; nights
can be cool even in the tropics.
- Do not be tempted to swim, as sharks
may be in the shade under the raft.

You may be too weak to re-board the raft.

- Attach the sea anchor at the liferaft entrance to benefit from any breeze.
- Keep as still as possible.
- Stay in any shade; cover head, neck and exposed areas.
- Use sunscreen and sunglasses, especially the lookout.
- Remember, reflection from the water can also cause sunburn.

Cold and wet

In cold climates it is vitally important to try to keep as warm and dry as possible.

- Remove wet clothing, wring out and put back on.
- Distribute spare dry clothes.
- Keep the raft as dry as possible.
- Adjust the openings for the minimum ventilation.
- Huddle together for mutual warmth but do not upset the trim of the raft.
- Sit on something to protect against the cold water. Use a lifejacket to sit on in calm seas, but wear the lifejacket in rough conditions.
- Use TPAs as they will reflect back 90 per cent of the body heat; feet will remain dry even in a partly water-filled liferaft.

Allocate TPAs to the coldest crew first; if two can fit in one bag, bundle a warmer person with a cold individual.

Once warm, open up the top layer of clothing, so body warmth acts like a radiator to keep the whole raft cosy. Stretch limbs, wriggle toes and fingers, to maintain blood circulation and avoid cold injury.

In very cold conditions, rotate the lookout watch at frequent intervals.

Decide on food and water rations

At best, your liferaft emergency pack will have 1.5l (0.4 gallons) of water per person; at worst, none at all.

The minimum daily amount of water considered necessary to survive in good shape is:
- 1l (0.25 gallons) in the tropics.
- 0.5l (0.1 gallons) in temperate climates.
- 55–220cc (2–5oz) for a short period.

The emergency food rations, if available, should be divided:
- 100–125gm (3–4oz) per person per day.
- Distribute at the same time as the water ration.

Unless fresh water is plentiful and you know rescue is on the way, divide the agreed ration thus:

First day: No water or food, except for the sick, injured, near drowned or very young.

Second day and thereafter: Agreed ration divided into three servings.

Last day minus one: Half the normal ration.

Regardless of how soon you expect to be rescued:

- Collect all rainwater.
- Start making water with a handheld water maker immediately.
- Use made water and any from the yacht first. The water in a liferaft pack will keep indefinitely.
- Do not eat anything unless you can also have a drink.

- Do not drink urine; it can kill you.
- The general rule is do not drink seawater (see Chapter 7).

Issue food and water at set times each day to give everyone something to look forward to. sunrise, midday and sunset make good times. Cut foil water pouches with scissors as tearing risks losing precious water. For morale, rations must be seen to be issued fairly; a minimum daily water ration should be 0.5l (0.1 gallons) more for the injured. Water should be swilled round the mouth before swallowing slowly.

Food rations should be distributed to last as long as possible. Do not eat anything caught unless 1l (0.25 gallons) of water can be drunk per day.

Take measures to maintain morale

Morale and the will to survive are very important. Morale will probably be lowest about three hours after abandoning your yacht. Seasickness, anxiety, extreme cold and the absence of food or water will further lower morale. Always make sure that ration issues are fair and on time.

Keep peoples' minds focused on eventual rescue and attracting attention; never talk of defeat or death in the liferaft. Use anything and everything to keep everyone cheerful including competitions, card games, songs and jokes. Listen to commercial broadcasts if you have a radio.

People with a strong will to survive can overcome seemingly impossible difficulties.

Make sanitary arrangements to keep the liferaft habitable

To avoid problems everyone should:
- Attempt to urinate within two hours of boarding the raft.
- Attempt a bowel movement within the first 24 hours.
- In calm seas, rig a safety line to aid defecation and urination over the side.
- In rough seas, use a bailer, bucket or other receptacle.
- Use the special sick bags from the liferaft pack, the dog poo bags packed in your grab bag or any other plastic bag – wash out and reuse them.
- Clean up all waste and throw it over the side immediately.
- If sharks are around, be careful about disposing of anything over the side.

Maintain the liferaft including topping up of buoyancy tubes and canopy supports

It is important to your survival that the liferaft is kept in good condition. A properly inflated liferaft is less likely to wear. Use plugs in top-up valves when not in use.

In hot weather, remove plugs regularly to allow excess pressure to escape and

 Remember: *No one is a survivor until they have been rescued.*

ensure adequate ventilation to avoid a build-up of carbon dioxide.

At night and on cooler days, top-up soft buoyancy tubes and canopy supports.

Make proper use of available survival equipment

Everyone must understand:

- How to use all equipment, especially signalling devices.
- The importance of all the search and rescue equipment for ultimate rescue.
- The potential to damage the raft with equipment, such as pyrotechnics.
- The necessity of preserving every item in perfect condition and inside the liferaft, by returning it to the stowage position or fastening it to themselves or the liferaft by means of a lanyard.

Prepare actions for arrival of rescue units, being taken in tow, rescue by helicopter and landing and beaching

Everyone aboard the liferaft, especially the lookout, must be ready for the possible arrival of SAR units or the sighting of land. Rescue can arrive by air as well as by sea. The ocean is large and a liferaft very small and hard to see, especially in rough weather. Proper use of any or all of the signalling equipment will help attract attention. See Chapter 10 for more information.

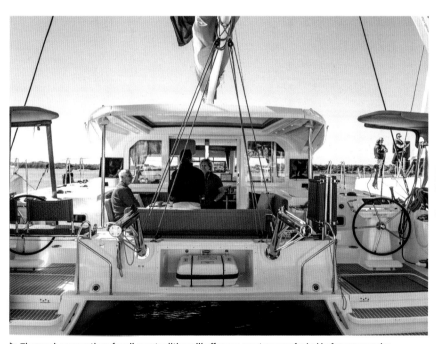

▶ Thorough preparations for all eventualities will offer you great peace of mind before your cruise.

7 LONG-TERM SURVIVAL IN A LIFERAFT

WITH GOOD COMMUNICATION equipment on board your yacht, and an EPIRB or two in your liferaft, this chapter is probably superfluous. Unfortunately, as they say, 'the best laid plans of mice and men….' and there are still wild and lonely places in the world where few others sail. The SAR authorities may be on their way; a fixed wing aircraft may sight you, but rescue by helicopter or boat may be delayed.

As the hours pass, it is essential to keep up morale and to always maintain a vigilant lookout. Good liferaft management should continue right up to the moment you leave the liferaft. As the days pass without rescue, water and food will become increasingly important and it may be necessary to move the liferaft.

▶ Water

Water is essential for long-term survival. If rescue does not arrive quickly, what water you have aboard quickly becomes depleted, so where and how much more can be acquired becomes the priority. A healthy person can live without water for 7–10 days and without food for 20–30 days in temperate conditions. The body naturally loses water: 50 per cent as urine; 25 per cent as water vapour during respiration; 25 per cent as sweat. You also lose water as a result of seasickness and digestion. By reducing the amount of water the body loses, you reduce the amount you need.

Reduced urine

By not drinking water for the first 24 hours in the liferaft, the body's automatic response to reduced water intake will initiate reduced urine production.

Reduced respiration and sweat

Practise all the points included in Chapter 6, under 'Protect against heat'. The less you move, particularly in the tropics, the less water you will sweat out or expel in respiration.

If your liferaft has no canopy, create shade using whatever you have available such as oars, blankets and clothes. Pay special attention to protection for the lookout.

Reduced seasickness

Vomiting leads to both dehydration and exhaustion, and must be avoided at all costs. Use all the measures discussed in Chapter 6, under 'Issue anti-seasickness medicine'. If possible, take anti-seasickness pills during the first storm, especially if sea conditions were calm earlier. Do not eat if you feel sick.

Drinking urine

Urine contains poisonous waste products which the body has already discarded. It is of no use and urine must not be drunk. At best, your body will have to get rid of the waste again and this will take more water. Do not believe anyone who suggests someone else's urine is acceptable; they are lying, and it is just as bad for you as for them.

Drinking seawater

Drinking seawater is considered dangerous and will result in kidney failure. The salt in seawater must be dissolved using water from the body so that the kidneys can pass the salt into the urine. This sets up a vicious circle; the more salt water is drunk, the more fresh water is taken from the body cells to dissolve the salt.

In the 1950s a Frenchman, Dr Alain Bombard, experimented with drinking seawater and the French Navy then consequently undertook further research. The hypothesis that it is possible to drink small amounts of seawater under certain conditions is not supported by any other more recent research. In conclusion, the accepted advice is don't drink seawater.

Supplementing the water ration

The importance of supplementing water rations cannot be overstressed. Rationing is uncomfortable; saliva will disappear, lips will crack and you will feel weak. If delirium starts, this is a sign that more water is urgently needed to sustain life. A

watermaker (a manually operated reverse osmosis water pump) is, after the EPIRB, the most valuable item aboard your liferaft. Start to make water as soon as you get in the liferaft and use this water first, reserving the supplies in the raft and those you brought with you. Your next most likely source of fresh water comes from rain, followed by ice and condensation.

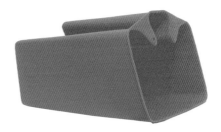

▶ A lifeboat bailer can be used to store water.

Collecting rainwater

Depending on location, rain can occur daily, occasionally or rarely. Unless rain is a daily occurrence, it is very important to be ready to take advantage of it. Lookouts must alert everyone to impending rain.

Leave rain-catching equipment ready before nightfall as sleepiness and darkness may make it harder to take advantage of a short rain shower. At the first sign of rain, remove salt crystallised over catchment areas by washing with seawater.

Use any large piece of fabric, such as sails, large plastic bags, heavy weather gear etc, to catch rain. Cans and bottles make good containers but not good collectors. Some liferaft canopies have drainage tubes leading inside, through which rainwater can be directed into containers.

Keep catching equipment out of the sea to prevent contamination. However, in rough seas it may be impossible to collect uncontaminated fresh water.

Use every available container for storage – buckets, bailer, plastic bag etc. Keep the first water collected separately as it will probably contain a little salt. Use to clean wounds or sores and wash your skin. If rainfall persists and every container is full, use the excess for personal hygiene.

Drink rainwater slowly to prevent vomiting if you are on strict rationing.

Collecting ice

In the polar regions ice of various kinds is available:

- Old ice, a year or more old, will be free or nearly free of salt. Old ice is bluish, has rounded corners and splinters easily; new ice is grey, milky and hard.
- Water from icebergs is fresh, but they are dangerous to approach and should only be viewed as a source of fresh water in an emergency.
- If it is very cold, freeze seawater in containers. Salt will freeze last and concentrate in the middle. Then break ice from the sides only to get low saline water.
- Collect any ice off the surface of various pieces of equipment; it is fresh water, frozen condensation.

Other water sources

In dry places with little rain, night time brings copious condensation. Water may condense under the liferaft canopy or exposure cover. Keep some sponges or cloths separately and use only to collect this water.

Some parts of fish contain fresh water. Cut in half and drink the spinal fluid. You can also suck the liquid from the eyes of large fish.

Do not drink any other body fluids; they are rich in proteins and fat and will use more water to digest than you can gain from the fluid.

Solar stills and desalting tablets are included in some liferafts. Set up a solar still as soon as possible. They are slow to produce water and will only work when it is sunny and on calm seas.

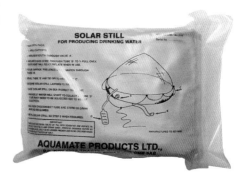

▶ An inflatable solar still.

Using foul water

Foul water is usually safe to drink but it may be so unpalatable that it causes retching. Up to 0.5l (0.1 gallons) can be absorbed rectally using an enema. In severe dehydration, an enema is often the best way of rehydrating the body. Do not use salt water for this purpose; it is as dangerous rectally as orally.

▶ *Food*

The digestion of food requires a lot of water; do not eat if you cannot drink. Over a short period you can survive without food. Over a long period you need to eat for energy and health. Protein requires more water to digest than carbohydrates. Since everything you are likely to catch contains protein, do eat anything caught without at least 1l (0.25 gallons) water per day. If water supplies are low, eat survival craft rations, which are specially designed to require little water. Also eat carbohydrates such as sugars and starches. Do not eat proteins or anything dried.

Very little waste residue results from eating emergency rations, so do not worry if you become constipated; this will also prevent the loss of valuable body water.

Supplementing the food ration

If fresh water is plentiful, eat any food brought or caught from the vessel, before using liferaft emergency rations. The sources of additional food at sea are limited to fish, birds, seaweed, turtles, shellfish and possibly plankton. With adequate water, the sea can provide enough food to sustain life for a long time. Eating fish alone may cause vitamin deficiencies, so if you have multivitamin tablets in your grab bag take them regularly. With ingenuity, most of what is around you in a liferaft can be used to catch, attract or find food.

Catching fish

Fish are plentiful in most oceans and can be caught relatively easily; flying fish may even throw themselves at you. If you cannot or do not want to eat the fish you catch for some reason, such as other available food or lack of water, still continue to fish as this can act as a morale booster and it never hurts to practise a skill that may, in time, be needed to sustain life.

Improvisation can turn several items into fishing equipment, for example:
- Line from unravelled threads or rope.
- Hooks from metal, plastic etc.
- Lures from any shiny metal, feathers, the intestines of an earlier catch etc.
- A spear from a knife tied very securely to an oar.
- A gaff from your largest hook attached to an oar.

It is very easy to damage an inflatable liferaft so be careful with anything sharp, such as hooks and spears. Fish can jump and harm the liferaft, as well as disappearing over the side. Do not try to land anything too large; better to go hungry than end up swimming because the raft has sunk.

Fishing equipment is very easy to lose so tie everything very carefully. If possible, include a line back to the raft or held by another person. Do not throw a spear that has your only knife attached to it.

Line fishing
Use small fish as a lure to catch bigger relatives, and keep bait moving in the water so it looks alive.

Spear fishing
Throw the spear straight down into the water, not at an angle, to avoid refraction errors. Once spiked, land fish quickly to prevent it slipping back off the blade. Tie the eye of the hook to the raft in case the hook comes off the shaft.

Gaffing

Put the gaff in the water, hook upwards, and wait for a fish to swim by. Aim for the stomach and get the fish straight on board as fast as possible.

Speargun fishing

A proper speargun is by far the easiest method of catching fish; you use it in the same way as a spear. Be very careful as you bring it back aboard the raft so as not to tear it. Spearguns can be used to land or kill large fish caught by line.

Attracting fish

By day, fish may be lurking under the raft, attracted by the shade. By night, use an electric light or try reflecting the light of a full moon using a signalling mirror.

Flying fish are found in schools and a light will attract them. Hold a light-coloured sheet vertically, even during the day; as they fly over the fish will hit it and fall stunned into the raft, in theory at least.

Using your catch

Most fish caught in the open sea are likely to be edible. Healthy fish can safely be eaten raw; it is a delicacy in many countries, and you can eat everything except the intestines.

Poisonous fish are usually found in coastal areas, particularly reefs. The dangerous types have spines, spikes, bristles or puff themselves up. Some can be eaten if the internal organs are discarded but, like eating toadstools and mushrooms, do not attempt it unless you are sure. If you must eat poisonous fish to survive, only eat flesh that has not been in contact with organs and do not touch the spines with bare hands.

Eat a small amount, wait a few hours for any adverse reactions, then eat more.

Fish should be gutted and bled as soon as possible after catching. In hot weather eat within half a day or dry, especially dark meat. Never eat fish with pale, shiny gills, sunken eyes, flabby skin or flesh, or an unpleasant odour. Good fish are the opposite of the above and have a saltwater or clean fishy odour.

To dry fish, or anything else caught, hang up fillets in the sun or cut into thin slices and lay out in the sun. High humidity can make it hard to dry food successfully.

When eating dried fish or meat, you should only consume with a plentiful supply of water. Check very carefully to make sure it is not rotten and if green or slime develops, scrap off and redry. If the flesh is disintegrating throw it away. Left over fish, or anything doubtful, can be used as bait.

Birds

All sea birds are edible although the taste may not be attractive and they can take a lot of chewing. They can be caught most successfully by hand, hook, spear or snare. If a bird lands on your raft for a rest, grab it quickly and wring its neck.

The easiest way to catch a bird is with a hook and line. Attach fish or meat to the hook and float it on the water; when the hook is taken pull in the line.

To spear a bird, place a bit of cloth or bright metal on the water near the raft. When the bird lands, throw the spear (attached to a line).

To snare a bird, make a large lasso from rope that will float. Spread out the loop on water, holding the end of the rope. Place a bit of cloth or bright metal in the centre of noose, then when the bird lands tighten the noose.

Using your catch
- Skin a bird and eat everything, except the intestines.
- Break the bones to extract the marrow.
- Entrails, feet and feathers can be used as bait.
- Fat under the bird's skin can lubricate your skin.
- In cold weather feathers can be used as insulation and fat is a valuable food.

Seaweed

Most seaweeds are edible although salty. They are a good source of protein, vitamins, minerals and fibre. You must have water to rinse and drink with seaweed. If you do not have enough, collect the seaweed and dry it to await sufficient water. Even if the seaweed is too tough to eat raw, carefully inspect every bit that passes the raft for small fish or crabs that can be eaten.

Plankton

Plankton is very nutritious and will be found in any area where whales live. It is easiest to collect at night when it is near the surface. It looks like grey scum and is best mixed with something else, but it will provide valuable protection from scurvy. A towed net is needed to collect plankton and ideally a speed of about 2 knots. A specially made net is best, but you can improvise with any material, and a spare sea anchor makes a perfect plankton net.

Barnacles

Without any antifouling, your liferaft will soon grow barnacles and in a few weeks, they will be big enough to eat. These will also grow on any lines trailing in the water and will be easier to get at than those under the raft. Eat barnacles whole; the shell also provides nutrition.

▶ Protection

If the time aboard the liferaft is measured in days rather than hours, it becomes even more important to take care of your delicate vessel. Unlike a yacht, rafts are manufactured for just days of use, rather than years. Wear is the biggest problem, and any line or object that touches an inflatable raft has the potential to eventually wear a hole. It is important to try to prevent this by padding and changing their position.

Outside the raft, problems may come from sea creatures underneath. As the time in the water increases, rafts without antifouling are susceptible to weed and barnacles and these are attractive to turtles, fish and sharks. While anything touching the raft is frightening, this may have a positive side, such as an opportunity to catch dinner.

Sharks

Sharks are creatures that invoke fear in most sailors, despite the softer picture projected by recent nature films. There are sharks in every ocean, and while many live and feed in the depths, others hunt near the surface. When you are in the liferaft and see sharks:

- Do not throw anything overboard by day; wait until it is dark.
- Do not fish and if you have hooked a fish, discard it.
- Do not let arms, legs or equipment hang in the water.
- Make sure everyone keeps quiet and still.
- Do not attempt to kill a shark for food, except as a last resort; they are very difficult to land without damaging oneself or the liferaft. Do not bring a shark the raft until it is dead. Cut off the head and skin immediately. Do not eat the liver as it is poisonous.

If a shark attack is imminent, hit it with anything except your hands. Be careful not to break or lose the article you use.

Heavy weather

Weather watching must not be limited to seeking rain clouds to supplement drinking water. It is also important for the lookout to be alert to any worsening conditions that could be a serious danger. It is also important that everyone is ready for the rough time ahead and that:

- Lifejackets are worn.
- Anti-seasickness tablets are taken.
- Sea anchors are deployed, and a second anchor prepared for use.
- All equipment is stowed or tied on with lanyards.
- Entrances are closed to prevent water entering.

- Crew are evenly distributed around the liferaft, with backs against the tubes and feet into the centre.
- If the liferaft is not full, crew should sit to windward to aid stability.

In very rough conditions, a second sea anchor can be streamed. If this is necessary, ensure the drogues' lines are of different length to prevent fouling.

▶ *Location*

In the past, the decision to stay at the scene of the sinking or to try to move

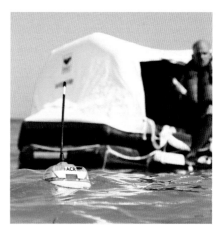

▶ Satellite equipment makes it likely that help is on the way.

away was more debatable. Now, with modern communications, particularly satellite equipment, making it likely that help is on the way, it rarely makes sense to move, even if it were possible to 'sail' a liferaft. Strong currents may move the raft rapidly away from the wreck, and if the wind is favourable it may be possible and sensible to sail back to the position of the disaster. It is important to remember that if a Mayday was sent from the vessel and not answered, that does not mean it hasn't been heard, and the centre of the search will always be the yacht's last position.

Once in the liferaft, the best method of communicating distress is an EPIRB. If the unit ceases to function before rescue is achieved, SAR authorities will use its last known position as the focus of the search area. If you have no EPIRB, or it is not working and you did not manage to make a distress call, an attempt to move away from the scene might be valid if:

- The vessel has sunk, and all possible useful items have floated to the surface.
- No one ashore will miss you and you did not leave a Voyage Details Plan.
- If five days have passed without help arriving.
- There is land, a shipping separation zone or an area frequented by fishing boats nearby.
- The wind and/or current is in the right direction.
- There is very little water and no rain expected.
- It is possible to 'sail' the raft.

Any decision to move away must be discussed and good reasons given to the crew to ensure their support, which is vital to the success of the venture.

Moving a liferaft

Sailing a liferaft is difficult because they are not designed to do this. One manufacturer does make a sailing liferaft, but it is a dinghy first and a liferaft second. Current and wind will affect the liferaft's progress – a portable GPS will be very helpful in monitoring this movement. With the sea anchor rigged:

- The current is the main influence on the movement of a liferaft
- The lower the raft is in the water, the greater the effect.
- Ordinary liferafts do not have keels and cannot be sailed into the wind. Therefore, direction of travel will be downwind, or slightly off that, otherwise there is no point in attempting to rig a sail.

If you do decide to sail, ensure the liferaft is fully inflated; take in the sea anchor, use an oar as a rudder and rig a sail and/or experiment with the liferaft openings.

If you decide to head for land, unless it is in sight, choose a land target that is large – the larger the better, ideally a continent. A small island may be near but is all too easy to miss. When land is in sight, use any onshore wind in the mornings and possibly the afternoons. Use the sea anchor at night to stop an offshore breeze pushing you away.

If you need water, the longer wind travels over water, the more vapour it will pick up. Downwind is usually the direction towards rain in the middle of the ocean.

▶ Psychological Disintegration

As time passes in a liferaft it is all too easy for psychological problems to increase just as easily as the physical problems of surviving. Denial can lead to apathy, apathy to depressed reaction, depressed reaction to despair and despair to psychological disintegration. Once that final stage is reached death is not far away.

The initial symptoms include irritability, sleep disturbance and mild startle reaction. Later comes social withdrawal, loss of interest, apprehension, general mental and physical retardation, confusion and finally death. Death, when it comes, can be a passive sinking or it can suddenly be considered a serious option, with suicide an easier alternative to the struggle to live. This breakdown can happen to an individual but can also affect a group. It can develop progressively or a particular event can act as a sudden trigger.

One common event that can severely upset survivors in a liferaft is to watch a potential rescue craft fail to sight the raft and then turn away. At such times, a strong leader may be all that keeps a group functioning and fighting on. A fierce determination to live, the willingness to improvise and regular activity, both mental and physical, can overcome most things. Water and food may be scarce but they can be found in most areas, and with rationing life can go on. The strengths of each member of the group add to that of the others and increase the chance for everyone to reach the ultimate goal of rescue and survival.

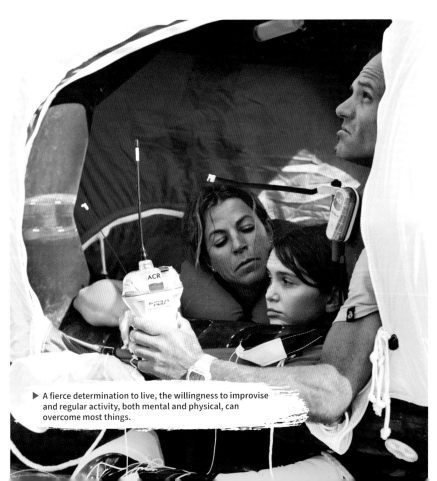

▶ A fierce determination to live, the willingness to improvise and regular activity, both mental and physical, can overcome most things.

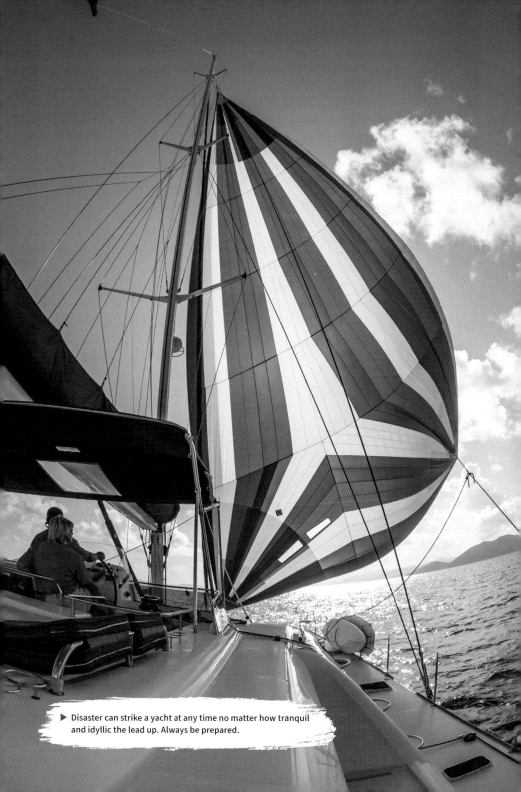

▶ Disaster can strike a yacht at any time no matter how tranquil and idyllic the lead up. Always be prepared.

8 INITIAL FIRST AID AND EMERGENCY TREATMENT

A first aid kit is supplied with some liferaft packs. Hopefully, you will also have brought the medical box from your yacht. This section provides basic information on emergency treatment of injuries and other immediate medical problems that may need to be dealt with aboard a liferaft.

▶ General Assessment

WITH ANY PATIENT, it is important to make a rapid examination to assess responsiveness and the extent of the injury:

- If the patient is unconscious, go straight to the 'Unconsciousness' section.
- If there is serious bleeding, go to the 'Bleeding' section.
- Handle the patient as little and as gently as possible so as to prevent further injuries and further shock.
- Place the patient in the most comfortable position possible and loosen tight clothing so that they can breathe easily.
- Do not remove more clothing than is necessary and be as gentle as possible.
- With an injured limb, get the sound limb out of the clothing first then peel the clothes off the injured limb,

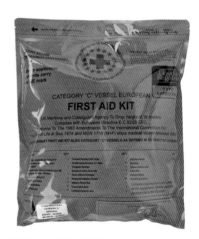

▶ A Category 'C' first aid kit.

which should be supported by another person during the process.

Shock can be a great danger to life, especially in the case of liferaft survivors, and one of the main objects of first aid is to prevent this.

Once it has been established that there is no immediate threat to life, there will be time to decide what treatment is possible in the liferaft. It is very important to be reassuring and compassionate, even though there may be little that can be actively done to provide a cure.

▶ Unconsciousness

The immediate threat to life may be:
- Breathing obstructed by the tongue falling back and blocking the throat.
- Stopped heart.

> It is important to remember the ABCs:
> **A** is for Airway
> **B** is for Breathing
> **C** is for Circulation

A is for Airway

This means establishing an open airway, by tilting the forehead back so that the casualty can breathe easily.

1 Lay the casualty flat on their back.
2 Place your hand on the casualty's forehead.
3 Place the fingers of your other hand under their chin.
4 Tilt their head and lift the jaw.
5 Open their mouth and remove any obvious obstructions such as blood, vomit or secretions, with your fingers or a clean piece of cloth.

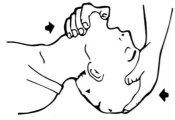

▶ Opening the airway.

6 Only remove any dentures if they are broken or displaced.

These actions may relieve the obstruction to breathing. The casualty may gasp and start to breathe naturally. If so, go on to the 'Recovery position' section.

B is for Breathing

Check for breathing – Look/Listen/Feel for three to five seconds:
- **Look** for movements of the chest and abdomen.
- **Listen** for breathing with your ear over the mouth and nose.
- **Feel** for the patient's breathing on your cheek.
- **Note** the colour of face and lips – normal or blue/grey tinge?

Not breathing

Begin **artificial respiration** at once – seconds count. **Never give rescue breathing to a person who is breathing normally.**

1 Check the airway remains open using head tilt and chin lift.
2 Move to one side of the patient.
3 Pinch the casualty's nose with your finger and thumb. After taking a full breath, seal your lips about the patient's mouth and blow into their mouth for about two seconds, until you see the chest rise.
4 If a barrier device is available, use it. In water, use mouth to nose.
5 Give two effective inflations quickly, then note if the colour of the face and lips is improving.

If there is improvement, continue the artificial respiration, at a rate of about 12 inflations each minute (count to five, slowly, between inflations). When the patient commences breathing go on to the 'Recovery position' section. If there is no improvement:

• Listen for heart sounds.
• Feel the pulse in the neck.
• Check for any coughing or movement of the chest.

If no heartbeat is found, the heart has stopped; begin **CPR** at once. You have at best, four to six minutes to restore circulation.

C is for Circulation and CPR (cardio-pulmonary resuscitation)

The casualty must be on a hard surface for CPR to be effective, which may be difficult in a liferaft.

1 Kneel, facing the casualty's chest.
2 With your fingers, locate the lower edge of the ribcage on the side closest to you.
3 Slide your fingers up the ribcage to the notch at the end of the breastbone.
4 Place your middle finger on the notch, and your index finger next to it.
5 Place the heel of your other hand on the breastbone next to your index finger.
6 Place the heel of the hand used to locate the notch on top of the heel of your other hand, interlocking the fingers if desired.
7 Position your shoulders over your hands, with elbows locked and arms straight.
8 Press firmly to produce a downward movement of about 4cm (1.5–2in). Repeat rapidly, at the rate of 80–100 times a minute.

9 Artificial respiration must be continued when giving heart compression since breathing stops when the heart stops.
  • With one person: 15 compressing thrusts, then two deep breaths
  • With two people: give five compressions and one deep inflation on the upstroke of the fifth compression.

Check for response: if the heart starts to beat, the colour of the face and lips will improve and the eye pupils will get smaller. Listen again for heart sounds and feel for a neck pulse after one minute and then at three-minute intervals. If they are heard, stop heart compression but continue with artificial respiration until natural breathing is restored.

When you are satisfied that the heart is beating and the patient is breathing naturally, carry on to the 'Recovery position' section.

Even in a fully equipped hospital with a team of trained doctors, CPR is not always successful. Attempting CPR can do no further harm; the patient is dead if you do not make an attempt. Try to continue the process for at least one hour. Never consider anyone to be dead until you and anyone else in the liferaft agrees that:

• Breathing has stopped and cannot be restarted.
• No pulse is felt and no sounds are heard when your ear is put to the chest.
• The eyes are glazed and pupils are dilated.
• There is a progressive cooling of the body.

Recovery position

Place the casualty in the unconscious or recovery position to keep the airway clear.

- Turn patient onto one side.
- To keep the body in stable position, bend and pull up the leg and the arm on the side to which the head is facing.
- Pull up chin to give clear airway. Keep mouth downwards to avoid chocking. Stretch other arm out along the other side of the body.
- In the liferaft it may be necessary to wedge the patient in this position using lifejackets, and possibly lash them in place.
- Any carbon dioxide build-up in the liferaft will be very dangerous for an unconscious casualty. Watch carefully for any gas leaking from the buoyancy tubes and keep the raft well ventilated.

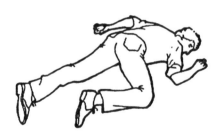

▶ Recovery position.

- Loosen clothing and remove any false teeth or spectacles.
- Do not give fluids or anything else to eat or drink.
- Treat for shock when the casualty regains consciousness.

▶ Near Drowning

Immediately treat any unconscious victims as described in the 'Unconsciousness' section. Immersion victims may vomit during or immediately after resuscitation, due to the amount of water they have swallowed and/or the inadvertent distension of the stomach, particularly if the neck was not well extended.

- Check the casualty's airway frequently to ensure that it remains clear.
- Do not try to drain water from the lungs of near-drowned victims.
- Give extra water rations as soon as they can drink to avoid dehydration.
- Casualty may also need to be treated for hypothermia.

Victims recovered from cold water near to drowning may show all the symptoms of death:

- Blue skin.
- No detectable breathing.
- No apparent pulse or heartbeat.
- Pupils wide open.

They may not be dead; the body may have gone into the mammalian diving reflex. For this to happen the water temperature must be less than 21°C (70°F), the face must have been immersed and the victim will probably be young.

Many children have been successfully resuscitated from freezing water after 30 minutes as the blood is diverted from the arms and legs to circulate between the heart, brain and lungs.

- Do not give up until the body has warmed up but still shows no sign of life.
- Give artificial respiration if hypothermia is suspected.
- Be sure all pulse is absent before you start CPR, see the 'Hypothermia' section.

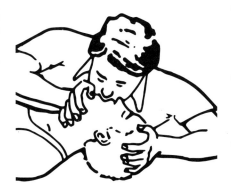

▶ Artificial respiration.

▶ *Bleeding*

Severe bleeding must be stopped as soon as possible. Action to be taken:

- Lay the casualty down.
- Clear away any clothing to expose the wound.
- Do not use a tourniquet.
- Press where the blood comes from, using a clean handkerchief, dressing or cloth, for 5–15 minutes.
- Do not remove anything embedded in the wound; instead, apply pressure beside the fragment.
- Press down hard with your hand or fist on the wound if nothing else is available. If possible, wear disposable gloves.

- If direct pressure is impossible, apply indirect pressure at a pressure point between the wound and the heart for a maximum of 15 minutes.
- Raise the bleeding part of the body to a near-vertical position if possible as this will help to stop the bleeding. Do not raise the limb if it is fractured.
- Bandage firmly around the wound to maintain the pressure, if necessary add more padding if bleeding continues.
- Keep the injured part as still as possible, and the casualty at rest, because movement will disturb and destroy blood clots.

This treatment applies equally to bleeding from an amputation site, when pressure should be applied over and around the end of the stump.

Do not attempt to remove any foreign objects in a wound unless they are superficial and can easily be removed.

Internal bleeding

If internal bleeding is suspected, lay the patient down with the feet raised, loosen clothing and treat them as for shock.

Chest wounds

A superficial chest wound should be treated as for any wound elsewhere. A penetrating wound, which makes a sucking sound, must be sealed immediately otherwise the lungs will not be able to inflate, as the vacuum inside the chest will be destroyed. Action to be taken:

- Temporarily plug the wound with the casualty's own bloodstained clothing.
- Cover the wound with a wet dressing, or use petroleum jelly on gauze.
- Seal on three sides only so the dressing acts as a one-way valve. As the patient breaths in, the dressing sucks down on the wound, and as they breathe out the air can escape through the flap valve.

The usual rules about stopping bleeding by pressing where the blood comes from also apply.

> Note: **Do not give morphine** to a patient with this type of wound, even if he is suffering from a lot of pain, because morphine will increase breathing difficulties.

Abdominal wounds

A superficial abdominal wound will require the same treatment as for any wound. For more serious wounds, take the following actions:

- If the abdominal contents do not protrude, cover the wound with a large standard dressing and place the casualty in the half-sitting-up position, or flat if the wound runs more or less vertically.
- If the abdominal contents do protrude through the wound, **do not attempt to put them back**. Cover with a loosely applied large standard dressing or dressings.
- Shock should be treated as below except:
  – Prop up if necessary.

– **Do not** give anything by mouth.
– If the patient is thirsty, moisten lips but nothing more.

▶ Shock

Shock is the result of, among other things, severe bleeding, injuries, burns, infections, heat exhaustion or lack of oxygen. The pulse becomes rapid and feeble; the skin is cold, clammy, and paler than normal, often greyish. Dizziness, fainting, vomiting and unconsciousness can occur. The state of collapse is due to a reduction in the volume of blood circulating in the body, caused by loss of blood, serum or fluids. Treat shock as follows:

- Stop the bleeding.
- Loosen clothes.
- Relieve pain.
- **Do not** give morphine when patient has breathing difficulties or severe head injuries.
- Cover with extra clothing but do not overwarm, especially if a lot of blood has been lost.
- Unless there are breathing difficulties, raise the legs of conscious patients.
- Reassure and encourage the patient.
- Be prepared to give artificial respiration and CPR.
- Place unconscious victim in recovery position.

▶ Hypothermia

Hypothermia is the term given to the condition when the deep body temperature is lowered below 35°C (95°F) and body functions become impaired. The rate of heat loss in water is many times greater than in air, and will vary depending on the difference in temperature between the body and the water. Any time spent in the water is likely to produce some degree of hypothermia. Heat loss will occur in any water below 35.5°C (96°F). In tropical water, death from hypothermia will take a considerable period, in colder waters it can occur in less than one hour.

Mild to Moderate Condition: 36–34°C (97–93°F)

The patient will suffer from:
- Shivering, cold hands and feet.
- Numbness in limbs, loss of dexterity, clumsiness.
- Irrational behaviour.
- Confusion, slurred speech.

Severe Condition: 33–29°C (92–84°F)

The symptoms change to:
- Shivering decreases or stops.
- Further loss of reasoning and recall, confusion and abnormal behaviour.
- Muscle rigidity develops.
- Skin becomes pale and pupils dilate.
- Pulse rate and breathing decreases.
- Victim semiconscious to unconscious.

Critical Condition: 28°C (82°F) and below

The patient's condition deteriorates:
- Breathing erratic and very shallow or may not be apparent.
- Victim is unconscious and may appear dead.

- Pulse slow and weak, or no pulse may be found.
- Skin is cold, may be bluish-grey in colour.
- The body is very rigid.

In a liferaft you should, if possible, actively treat hypothermia as follows:
- Gently strip off all wet clothing and replace with dry. Or wring out water and put back on.
- Use any spare clothing, blankets or TPAs for seriously affected victims.
- Huddle together under any covering to conserve heat and re-warm.
- Place seriously affected victims in close proximity to warmer survivors.
- Place a warm person in a TPA together with a hypothermic survivor.
- Use chemical heat packs in the armpits, groin and either side of the neck, before wrapping the victim up.
- Encourage the patient to urinate as body heat is wasted keeping urine warm.

But:
- **Never** rub or try to warm a hypothermic victim's limbs. This can send cold stagnant blood from the periphery to the core, further decreasing core temperature. It can lead to death.
- **Do not** give any alcohol or allow the patient to exert himself.

For severe hypothermic victims:
- Check breathing and heart rate very carefully.
- Be sure all pulse is absent before you start CPR. Premature cardiac massage may actually precipitate cardiac arrest.

- Start artificial respiration if breathing appears to be absent in order to increase available oxygen. Warm air blown into the lungs will also assist internal re-warming.
- Begin active re-warming, but do not remove clothes and avoid excessive handling of the casualty.

Do not give up resuscitation too soon. Casualties with hypothermia are never cold and dead, only warm and dead.

▶ Burns

All burns are serious, but if the burned area exceeds 10 per cent of the body surface, they are dangerous. Those exceeding 33 per cent of the body surface are often fatal. All burns create raw tissues susceptible to infection. The larger the area of body burned, the greater the shock and more seriously ill the patient.

Superficial (first degree) burns

These affect only the outer skin layers and cause reddening.
- Clean, if necessary, with fresh water.
- Leave open or cover with a clean dry dressing.

Moderate (second degree) burns

These cause reddening, blistering, swelling and weeping of fluids.
- Remove any constricting jewellery and clothing.
- Do not attempt to pull off any that are stuck.

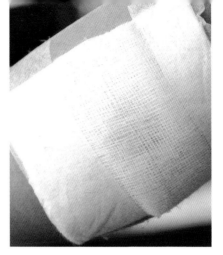

▶ All burns are serious, and if a burned area exceeds 10 per cent of the body surface, they are dangerous.

- Wash the area with soap and fresh water, using a lint-free cloth.
- Do not touch with your hands.
- Do not burst any blisters.
- Cover with a paraffin gauze dressing, then more gauze, cotton wool and a bandage.
- Loosen the dressing if swelling occurs.
- Do not disturb dressing for a week, unless it becomes very smelly, dirty or the patient's temperature is raised.
- Give the patient as much water as possible to replace lost body fluids.
- Treat for shock and administer pain medication.

Deep (third degree) burns

Deep burns will have destroyed all skin and may have penetrated to underlying fat, muscle and bone. There is little you can do for this condition, or any extensive burns, in a liferaft. Cover the area with clingfilm if available, and treat as for moderate burns.

▶ Fractures

Unless expert medical attention is available, little can be done for the patient in a liferaft except to immobilise the fracture with bandages, slings and splints.

- If nothing is available to make a splint, use the patient's own body, eg strap broken leg to whole one, use duct (elephant) tape with cloth or paper to stop it sticking to the skin. Do not strap so tightly that circulation is affected.
- Make the patient as comfortable as possible.
- Provide pain relief and treat them for shock.
- Prevent movement caused by rolling liferaft by placing patient between two fit survivors.

▶ Fuel Oil Contamination

Survivors who have spent time in water that has been contaminated by fuel oil are likely to be affected by:

Swallowing of oil

- Usually causes vomiting; the effect will wear off in a few days.
- Give milk or additional water to replace body fluid lost if vomiting.

Clogging of skin pores

- Oil on the skin should be cleaned off as much as possible.
- If totally smothered in oil, skin cannot perspire or breathe; this can kill.

Pollution of lungs

- Little can be done in the raft.
- It can be dangerous and lead to pneumonia.
- Rest, warmth and fresh air are about the only treatment.

Inflammation of the eyes

- Wash out with seawater.
- Protect from bright sunlight until any inflammation has gone.

Treat any wounds as if the oil was not present.

▶ Prescription Drugs

Be very cautious about taking any drugs while in the liferaft if water and food are in short supply. The way many drugs affect the body will be altered by dehydration. Be cautious about continuing to take regular medicines or courses of treatment started while aboard the yacht, unless not to do so would be life threatening.

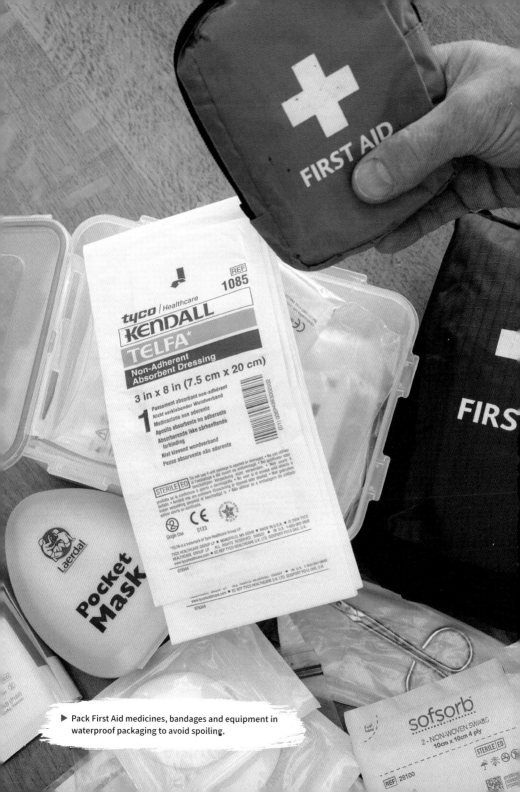

▶ Pack First Aid medicines, bandages and equipment in waterproof packaging to avoid spoiling.

9 FIRST AID FOR LIFERAFT AILMENTS

Living in a liferaft with little room and no real exercise is hard, even in perfect conditions where food and drink are plentiful, seas are calm and the weather is mild. In most cases, perfect conditions will not prevail and people will suffer, especially if rescue is long delayed.

▶ Seasickness

WHILE A FEELING of nausea is almost inevitable in a liferaft either at first or during the first storm, actual seasickness must be avoided if possible. Some people are always more susceptible than others, but most eventually get used to the movements of a vessel after a few days and suffer less. Seasickness can cause:

- Extreme fluid loss and exhaustion.
- Depression and the loss of the will to live.
- Others to become nauseated.
- Sharks to be attracted to the liferaft.
- Unclean conditions.

Various ideas for reducing seasickness have been discussed in Chapters 3 and 6, though for some people the only real cure is to 'sit under a tree' – get off the liferaft.

Treatment for seasickness

- Wash the patient and the liferaft to remove the sight and smell of vomit.
- Do not give the patient any food until the nausea has gone.
- Flat cola type drinks may be helpful in settling the stomach and rehydrating.
- Lay the patient down for rest, covered with warm coats or blankets.
- Give the patient anti-seasickness pills rectally if possible.
- Use prescription anti-emetic, unless the patient is pregnant.

▶ Cold Injuries

All cold injuries are connected to the reduction of peripheral circulation, as the body attempts to reduce heat loss in the core. Various factors affect a person's susceptibility to cold injuries. Obviously low temperatures are needed but wind chill, wet skin, exposed skin, previous cold injuries, tight clothes, cramped position, body type, dehydration, calorific intake, diabetes and some medications can all be influences.

Frostbite

Watchkeepers or survivors in open liferafts are particularly prone to tissue fluids freezing in localised areas of the body. It usually occurs at the body's extremities – fingers, toes, ears, etc. The depth of damage is graded like burns into first degree (frostnip), second degree (superficial frostbite), third degree (severe frostbite) and fourth degree (deep frostbite). The signs are:

- Cold with pale to waxy white skin colour.
- Initial tingling and stiffness, changing to numbness and anaesthesia.
- Skin changes from hard, rubbery top layer to wooden all the way through.
- Finally, freezing of muscle and/or bone.

To reduce the risk of frostbite, all watchkeepers should:

- Wear protective clothing.
- Reduce lookout periods in very cold weather and watch each other's condition.
- Wriggle nose and checks, and exercise hands and feet to keep circulation going.
- Not smoke, as this reduces peripheral blood circulation.

At the first sign of frostbite, immediate steps should be taken to re-warm the frozen parts and to get out of the wind.

- Do not massage affected area once signs of frostbite have appeared.
- Warm area by:
  - Blowing warm air on it.
  - Holding a hand against it.
  - Placing hands under armpits etc.

In theory, if you cannot guarantee that the tissue will stay warm, third and fourth degree frostbite should not be re-warmed. Once the tissue is frozen, harm has already been done and keeping it frozen will not cause significant additional damage. On the other hand, refreezing after warming can cause extensive damage and may result in loss of tissue. On a liferaft, unless help is nearby, you probably do not have much choice.

If a person is hypothermic as well as frostbitten, the first concern is body core re-warming. Do not re-warm frostbitten areas until the body core is almost normal.

When treatment has been ineffective, skin dies and becomes black. If this occurs, dry dressings should be applied to the affected parts.

Chillblains

These are caused by repeated exposure of the skin to temperatures above freezing but below 16°C (60°F). Redness and itching affect the area and the skin swells and becomes bluish red. Chilblains are found particularly on cheeks, ears, fingers and toes of women and children. Warming by breathing on them may help, though itching may be made worse. Do not massage the area. The cold causes permanent damage to the peripheral capillary bed and the redness and itching will return with re-exposure.

Immersion foot (trench foot)

Immersion foot is similar to chilblains. It occurs when:

- Local tissue temperature of the limbs (usually feet) remains subnormal but above freezing for prolonged periods.
- Exposed in a liferaft for several days if the feet are wet and immobile.
- Cold and usually, but not necessarily, immersed in cold water.
- Feet are immobile for prolonged periods with tight footwear.

The affected part will be:

- White, numb, cold and slightly swollen.
- If untreated, the skin tissue begins to die. Circulation can be permanently impaired and tissue damage can ultimately cause the loss of the limb.
- Hot, red, swollen and very painful with returning warmth.

Do not rub the skin when re-warming.

Every effort should be made to prevent immersion foot:

- Keep the liferaft as dry as possible.
- Keep feet warm and dry.
- Regularly exercise knee and ankle joints.
- Loosen shoelaces and raise feet.

- Remove shoes, warm feet under the armpits of others, but outside their clothes.
- Use spare clothes and plastic bags to wrap feet.
- Use TPAs to keep feet dry, even with water in the raft.

▶ *Heat Illnesses*

In warm or tropical climates, excessive exposure to the sun and heat can cause extremely bad cases of sunburn and hyperthermia (or heatstroke). Heat illnesses are the result of elevated body temperatures due to an inability to dissipate the body's heat and/or a decreased fluid level. Three levels of heat illness are likely in survival craft: heat cramps, heat exhaustion and, most serious of all, hyperthermia, which can kill. See Chapters 6 and 7 for methods of keeping cool and protected in a liferaft in hot weather.

Heat cramps

Often these are the first warning of heat exhaustion, they are a form of muscle cramp brought on by exertion and insufficient salt due to sweating. Actions to take:

- Move the patient to the coolest part of the liferaft.
- Sponge with seawater.
- Unless fresh water is severely rationed, replace salt and fluid with a commercial rehydration solution or mix one tablespoon of seawater with 400ml (16 fl oz) fresh water (one part seawater to 64 parts fresh

water), and drink slowly over an hour.
- Stretch the affected muscle.
- Do not knead and pound as this may cause residual soreness.

Heat exhaustion

This occurs when fluid losses caused by sweating and respiration are greater than the body's internal fluid reserves. Lack of fluid causes the body to constrict blood vessels in the arms and legs. Signs and symptoms are:
- Sweating.
- Skin pale and clammy.
- Pulse fast and weak.
- Respiration rapid and shallow.
- Nausea and vomiting.
- Patient weak, dizzy, thirsty and possibly has blurred vision.

Treatment should be similar to that for fainting, plus rehydration and rest. Actions to take:
- Move the patient to the coolest part of the liferaft.
- Sit or lie patient with their feet raised.
- Sponge with seawater.
- Unless fresh water is severely rationed, replace salt and fluid with a commercial rehydration solution or mix one tablespoon of seawater with 400ml (16 fl oz) fresh water (one part seawater to 64 parts fresh water), and drink slowly over an hour.
- Monitor carefully and check that heat exhaustion does not become hyperthermia.
- Make the victim rest for at least a day.

Hyperthermia (heatstroke)

Hyperthermia is the opposite of but is similar to hypothermia, in that it affects the body's core temperature. Key factors:
- Caused by working in the heat.
- The body cannot lose heat fast enough when fluid levels are low.
- Core temperature rises, leading to unconsciousness and possibly death.
- It can happen quickly.
- A victim can die if untreated.

The signs and symptoms of hyperthermia are:
- Hot skin: This is the key sign. It may be dry, or wet if the victim has just moved from heat exhaustion.
- Skin pale with flushed feverish face.
- Pulse rapid and strong.
- Respiration rapid and deep.
- Severe headache, often with vomiting.
- Pupils may be dilated and unresponsive to light.
- Fainting, delirium or seizures.
- The patient may become comatose, especially if core temperature is above 41°C (105°F).

Efforts to reduce body temperature must begin immediately.
- Move the patient to the coolest part of the liferaft.
- Remove clothing.
- Sprinkle with seawater or cover extremities with wet blankets.
- Fan to increase air circulation and improve evaporation.
- Massage extremities vigorously to help propel cooled blood back to the core.

- Once cooled, stop active cooling and cover.
- Monitor carefully, it may be necessary to re-cool the victim several times before temperature stabilises.
- Unless fresh water is severely rationed, replace salt and fluid with a commercial rehydration solution or mix one tablespoon of seawater with 400ml (16 fl oz) fresh water (one part seawater to 64 parts fresh water), and drink slowly over an hour.
- Make the victim rest for at least a day.

▶ Salt-water Boils

These are caused by the skin becoming sodden with seawater over a period of days. Actions to take:

- Do not squeeze or burst boils.
- Flush with fresh water.
- Apply an antiseptic ointment.
- Keep boils clean, and cover with a dry dressing.
- Keep area as dry as possible to avoid chafing.

▶ Dry Mouth and Cracked Lips

This is a common problem when water is limited. Actions to take:

- Swill any water around mouth prior to swallowing.

- Suck a button (removed from clothing).
- Smear lips with cream or petroleum jelly to reduce cracking.

▶ Swollen legs

A common problem caused by long periods spent in a sitting position. It will subside without treatment after rescue.

▶ Constipation

Liferaft rations do not produce a lot of waste products for the body to expel, and bowel movements in consequence will not be as frequent as normal. Actual constipation is a common problem on a liferaft in the long term with a diet of fish and little water. Actions to take:

- If plenty of fresh water is available, seaweed will provide good roughage.
- Do not take a laxative, this will increase dehydration.

▶ Urine Retention

This can be dangerous, and everyone should be encouraged to urinate as soon as possible after they arrive in the liferaft, while the body is still hydrated. With water rationing, normal urine production will be much reduced, and urine will appear dark and smoky.

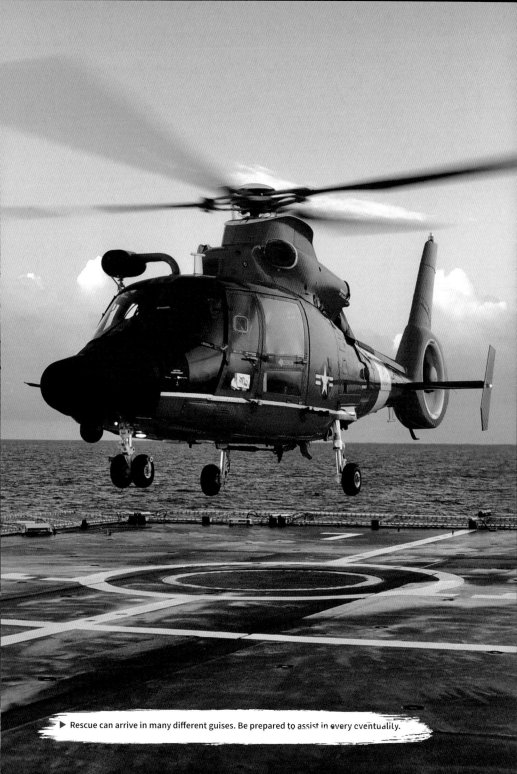

▶ Rescue can arrive in many different guises. Be prepared to assist in every eventuality.

10 RESCUE

IN THE MIDDLE of the Pacific Ocean, watchkeepers high up on the bridge of large ships will not be paying the same attention to looking for other yachts, let alone liferafts, unless they have already been alerted. While survival is necessary, rescue is the goal of everyone aboard a liferaft. If you contacted someone before the yacht sank, you know help is coming.

If an EPIRB was your only means of distress alerting, and the unit has good view of the sky, then the alert will be received almost instantaneously even without GPS. If the signal is partly obscured, for example if the unit was set off down below decks, there could be a delay. EPIRBs manufactured after 2022 will have a feature that shows the alert has been received by the authorities, a huge benefit over the earlier models that don't give this reassurance.

With no direct contact and no EPIRB, your chances of rescue depend upon:

- How far offshore you are.
- Whether you left a Voyage Details Plan with anyone.

Even in wartime, when lookouts were particularly alert, there were many occasions when ships failed to spot lifeboats and liferafts within easy distance, and even flares failed to attract attention. It is very difficult to spot a liferaft further than about 5 miles (8km) from the air by eye alone, on a fine sunny day, much less far from a ship in bad weather or poor visibility.

As soon as you know that help is in the area you should use all signalling equipment in the liferaft to indicate your position.

Once an aircraft or ship has been sighted, everyone in the liferaft will expect immediate rescue. This may not happen because a craft capable of recovering you might not be immediately available, or there may be a higher priority.

You must maintain survival routines until the moment of rescue.

Do not despair if you are not immediately sighted or if a crewmember mistakes a star, or the rising moon, for a ship. It is vital for your mental health and that of everyone else in the liferaft to remain optimistic. It can never hurt to include a prayer, to whichever deity you favour, for your safe deliverance.

▶ Who Might Arrive?

You should have some knowledge of SAR capabilities and procedures for the sea areas through which you are passing. Unfortunately, it is not always easy to get hold of this information for every area of the world.

SAR off the coasts of the UK

HM Coastguard, a division of the MCA, is the authority responsible for initiating and co-ordinating all civil maritime SAR measures for vessels in their search and rescue region. This is an area bounded by latitudes 45° and 61° North, by 30° West and by the adjacent European Search and Rescue Regions.

SAR off the coasts of the USA

The US Coast Guard (USCG) is responsible for initiating and co-ordinating all civil maritime SAR for vessels in their region. This is a huge area, and it includes the Caribbean and a large part of the northern Pacific Ocean.

The USCG handles most SAR operations themselves and can receive help from both the US Navy and the US Air Force when they request it. Close to the coast, the USCG is augmented by the USCG Auxiliary.

▶ Attracting the Attention of Rescue Units

Aside from any response to a satellite telephone conversation, a GMDSS alert or a signal acknowledgment on a modern EPIRB, the first indication of help at hand may be a message over your VHF, activation of the SART (Search And Rescue Transponder), sighting a craft or hearing an aircraft.

If you know rescue craft are in the vicinity it is important to use every means of attracting attention. Possible distances that a search vessel may receive your signal, assuming highest quality equipment and good conditions, are:

- EPIRB 121.5 MHz homing signal: Line of sight.
- EPIRB AIS signal: 4 miles (6.5km).
- Liferaft light on a SOLAS-compliant raft: 2 miles (3km).
- Flares (SOLAS):
  - Red parachute: 28 miles (44km).
  - Red handheld: 5 miles (8km).
  - Orange handheld smoke: 3 miles (5km).
  - Orange buoyant smoke: 6 miles (10km).
  - Electronic LED flares: 3–6 miles (5–10km).
- Radar reflector: Depends greatly on how high it is mounted.
- SART: 10 miles (16km).
- Signal mirror: 10 miles (16km).
- Signalling torch: 22 miles (35km).
- Strobe light: 5 miles (8km).
- VHF, handheld: 5 miles (8km).
- Whistle: Less than 1 mile (2km).

These distances may be much greater for SAR aircraft and will be reduced if the equipment is not of the best quality, or in bad weather with poor visibility.

Should you be lucky enough to be in contact by phone, cellular or satellite, this may not be enough to give rescuers your location. This is where you will be glad you had the forethought to install the free What3Words app on your phone. The app will give your current location, even if you don't have a phone signal or data connection. Of course, at sea on a moving liferaft, this will keep changing but should be accurate enough for the emergency services to roughly pinpoint your position. Be aware that the constant update of your location will drain your phone battery.

EPIRB

With rescue near at hand, your EPIRB should be attached outside the liferaft if it has a strobe light fitted, especially at night.

Pyrotechnics

Pyrotechnics flares should not be used unless it is certain that help is nearby. Remember that even modern electronic flares have a finite battery life. Do not look directly at any flare, electronic or otherwise, because its intense brightness may damage your vision, particularly at night.

Attracting attention

To attract attention, use a red parachute rocket:

- Fire slightly downwind; they are designed to turn into the wind.
- Aimed into the wind they may fail to gain altitude and be blown back aboard.
- With low cloud, fire about 45° downwind so it burns under the cloud.
- **Do not** fire when aircraft or helicopters are in the immediate area.

Pinpointing your position

Pinpoint your position when help is in sight with:

- Red handheld flares in poor visibility, high winds or darkness.
- Orange buoyant or handheld smoke flares in daylight, with good visibility and a light wind.

- Hold orange smoke and red handheld flares firmly downwind and clear of the raft, to prevent any hot ash hurting you or the liferaft.
- Throw a buoyant smoke signal into the water to leeward.

Signalling light

While it is almost impossible to use a heliograph to signal SOS in a liferaft, the same is not true with a torch. A regularly flashing light is more likely to be sighted, such as repeated flashing of SOS in Morse code, than simply shinning a torch in the direction of rescuers. Some electronic flares are preprogramed to flash the international SOS distress signal, which is three short flashes, three long flashes, and three short flashes. (•••---•••)

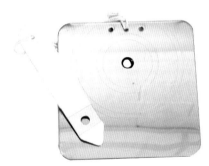

▶ Heliograph or signal mirror.

Signal mirror

A mirror is one of the most effective visual signals available in bright sunshine to attract attention. It is easiest to use when the sun is in the same direction as the target. Instructions for use should be included with the mirror:

- Raise the mirror close to your face.

- Sight the aircraft or vessel through the hole in the centre.
- Some sunlight should come through the hole and land on your face, or clothing.
- Tilt the mirror until the reflection disappears through the hole while still seeing the target.
- At that point, the sun will be reflected on the aircraft or vessel.
- The movement of the survival craft will provide sufficient flashing effect.
- Be careful not to blind the pilot of the aircraft.

VHF

If you have a portable VHF in your liferaft it will enable you to talk to your rescuers before they arrive. It can also be used by SAR units fitted with VHF direction finding equipment to locate the liferaft. A unit with DSC and AIS will also enable most commercial vessels to locate the liferaft accurately; a huge bonus as these vessels are unlikely to have VHF direction finding equipment.

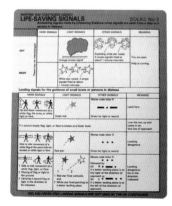

▶ SOLAS card with important signals.

Whistle

While the primary use of a whistle is for survivors in the water, both to attract their attention and for them to alert others to their position, it can also be used to indicate the position of a liferaft to searching vessels. This may be particularly important in restricted visibility when people are making a special effort to listen for any noise.

▶ The Arrival of Fixed Wing Aircraft

Fixed wing aircraft have a much greater range than helicopters and may be the first to find you. Unless you can alert overhead aircraft to your presence, they may consider their search to be a failure and move on to another area.

There are a few points to note:

- Use any means at your disposal to attract attention.
- Do not aim the flares directly at the aircraft, particularly helicopters; it will not help you if you endanger them!
- Use a portable VHF if you have one available; many rescue aircraft can be contacted using channel 16.

Fixed wing aircraft provide more than just verification that help is needed. They can:

- Provide an exact location of the distress to the shoreside authorities and ships in the vicinity.
- Guide rescue vessels and helicopters to the liferaft; invaluable in rough weather when wave heights are huge, and a small craft can be hard to spot.
- Keep the liferaft under observation and provide reassurance.

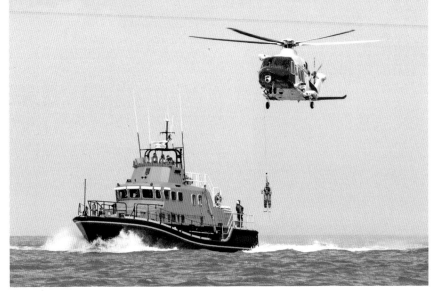

▶ A helicopter produces a very strong downdraft.

- Mark the position of the survivors with a sonobuoy (a radio beacon about 45cm (18in) long by 12cm (5in) in diameter, with a flotation bag and aerial on top) to help guide the rescue craft.

▶ Rescue by Helicopter

The ultimate in quick-fix rescues are those undertaken by helicopters. There are two main types of helicopters used for SAR in the UK; the Agusta Westland 189 and the Sikorski. These helicopters have an automatic hover control system and can effect rescues both at night and in fog where there are no visual hover references. The rescue can be dangerous, particularly in rough weather.

A helicopter produces a very strong downdraft; the raft and its occupants will receive a severe buffeting. Always follow the instructions of the helicopter crew, even if they differ from what you have learned in the past or what is written here.

- **Do not** touch the winchman, stretcher or winch hook until these have been earthed.
- **Do not** secure any lines passed down.
- Grab a line using a glove or cloth to prevent rope burn.
- Assist the winchman by pulling on the line as they approach liferaft.
- **Do not** fire parachute flares when a helicopter is in the area.
- **Do not** transmit on the radio while winching is in progress.
- **Do not** stand up, unless or until you have to.
- **Do not** shine a light at the helicopter at night.
- Tie down everything and remove any aerials, SARTs etc. Even a small piece of paper ingested into a helicopter engine can cause a crash.
- Don lifejackets unless this would cause unjustified deterioration to the condition of an injured person.
- Deploy the liferaft sea anchor.

- Remove any liferaft canopy if possible.
- Rebalance the raft as each person is winched out.

The skipper of the liferaft should liaise with the winchman to decide in which order the survivors should be evacuated. A special device for hoisting or lowering persons may be used and these are described below.

Rescue sling

This is the most common method of getting survivors into a helicopter. UK SAR helicopters always use a double lift where a winchman is lowered with a strop for a survivor. When there are several survivors to be rescued, the winchman may take two strops with them. In this case, when they reach the liferaft, the winchman will detach themselves from the winch hook and feed the survivors up to the helicopter two at a time.

If the winchman thinks survivors are cold and potentially hypothermic, they may elect to winch them in a horizontal position to minimise further injury. This is achieved with two strops, placing one under the armpits and the other behind the knees. If a single strop is supplied without a winchman, it must be used as follows:

1 Grasp the strop and put both arms and head through the loop.
2 Ensure the wide padded part is as high as possible across the back; the two sides are under the armpits and the wire is up in front of the face.
3 Pull toggle down as far as possible.

4 When ready, look up at the helicopter, put one arm out and give a clear 'thumbs up'.
5 Forget what you might have seen in the movies! Put and keep both arms down beside the body.
6 On being winched up alongside the helicopter, do nothing until instructed by the helicopter crew.

Other winch attachments

In some parts of the world it is more common to use an alternative to a rescue sling. One of the following may be attached to the end of the winch cable:

- *Rescue basket:* Climb into this, sit down and hold on.
- *Rescue net:* A conically shaped cage, open on one side; climb in, sit down and hold on.
- *Rescue litter:* Designed for hoisting injured survivors.
- *Rescue seat:* Can hoist two persons at once. It looks like a three-pronged anchor with flat flukes or seats. Sit astride one or two of the seats and wrap your arms around the shank.

▶ Rescue by Ship

If a ship is going to rescue you, it is important to clear away any lines, including the sea anchor and other gear, that could cause entanglement. Survivors must don their lifejackets, unless this could cause substantial deterioration in the condition of an injured person. The ship may approach so as to put the raft on its lee side and then drift down on you. Be careful of the raft being sucked into the propeller anywhere abaft the beam.

Alternatively, the ship may put a rescue craft or lifeboat into the water.

Boarding the ship may be by the liferaft being winched up with survivors aboard. You may have to climb aboard using ropes, a ladder or a scrambling net lowered over the side.

> Remember that after any period in a liferaft, survivors are likely to be weakened; do not overestimate strength, take extra care.

Preparation for being taken in tow

If the rescue craft is small, or the sea conditions are difficult, the liferaft may be towed to a place of safety before survivors are transferred. Actions to take:

- Use the painter or drogue line as a towline if they are in good condition.
- Attach a supplied line to the liferaft painter patch or bridle.
- Establish a simple communication system with the towing vessel.
- Pull in the sea anchor before towing commences.
- Once under way, remain as still as possible to keep the liferaft balanced.
- Watch out for chafe or damage to the liferaft during the tow.
- Keep a knife ready in case the towline needs to be cut in an emergency.

▶ Landing and Beaching

You might reach land rather than be rescued, and one of the watchkeeper's duties is to look carefully for any signs of land. There are many indicators that land

is near in addition to the obvious sighting on the horizon. They are:

- Drifting vegetation or wood.
- Birds (a single bird may be lost; repeated sightings may indicate nearby land).
- The direction flocks of birds fly at dawn and dusk. This may indicate the direction of land as some seabirds roost on land.
- Wind, which frequently blows towards land by day and away from land at night.
- Very light-coloured water. This indicates shallow water and nearby land. (Colour change only could be a continental shelf, hundreds of miles from land.)
- A greenish tint on the underside of a cloud layer in the tropics, is often caused by coral reefs or lagoons.
- Light-coloured reflections on the underside of a uniform cloud layer in the Arctic, may indicate ice fields or snow-covered land. (Open water reflects dark grey.)
- Fixed cumulus cloud in a clear sky, or where other clouds are moving. This often hovers over or slightly downwind of an island.
- A change in the pattern of the swell, which may indicate a change of tide around an island.
- A decrease in swell, while the wind remains constant. This may indicate an island to windward, protecting the sea.
- The sound of surf: this carries well over water, helpful at night, in fog, mist or rain.

- The smell of land; this can be very distinctive, especially after some time at sea.

Mirages can occur in any latitude, but they are more common in the tropics, especially in the middle of the day. Be careful not to mistake a mirage for nearby land. Try altering your position, standing up or sitting down, to check your sighting is real.

Landing

The greatest danger in any boat is not in the open ocean but near rocky or coral shores. Getting ashore safely in a liferaft is difficult, especially in anything but calm conditions. Take your time before making an attempting, and remember:
- A liferaft is hard to manoeuvre, easy to rip.
- The crew are probably not in peak condition.

The easiest landing will be:
- A flat sloping sandy beach.
- The lee side of an island.
- Inside a small bay that will shelter you from the waves.
- In day light.

If possible, avoid:
- Shores with high cliffs.
- Coral reefs.
- Breaking surf.
- Darkness.

If the shore looks unsuitable, try to paddle to a better place. Go around to the leeward side of an island and look for gaps in the surf line. Head for the mouth of a freshwater stream where there will not be any coral. If the coast is inhabited, try to attract attention before landing; the local inhabitants may be able to come out

to get you. Alternatively, they may direct you to a good landing spot. Unless it will clearly be an easy landing:
- Put on shoes, plenty of clothing and lifejackets to protect yourself from rocks and coral.
- Tie everything down to prevent it flying around.
- Hold on tightly, or use a safety line to attach yourself to the raft.
- Sit outside any canopy, to aid escape easily in the event of capsize.
- Consider cutting off the canopy, but keep it for use ashore.
- Waves often arrive in sets of seven; time your landing to coincide with the smallest one.
- Stream the sea anchor to avoid surfing and prevent a capsize.
- In heavy surf, consider filling the liferaft with water to make it more stable.
- Near surf, everyone should sit on the seaward side to maintain stability.

Approaching the shore

Paddle hard towards the beach between waves. Paddle back as hard as you can when the next breaking wave is catching you. If you are thrown out of the raft, hold on to the lifelines and stay with the raft as it is much more dangerous to swim ashore alone. Also, your liferaft contains all your supplies; they may be needed ashore.

If you seem to be drifting away from the shore it may be because you are caught in a rip current or the outflow of a river. Do not fight it, paddle across it, they are not usually very wide. Once clear, make for the shore.

As the raft nears the beach, try to ride in on the crest of a large wave. Paddle or row hard and ride the wave as far up the beach as possible. Do not jump out of the raft until it has grounded.

Once grounded, be quick to get out and beach your craft. Drag the raft above the tide line.

▶ Ashore

The priorities once everyone is safely ashore will depend upon where you are, the time of year and the condition of all the other crewmembers. Surviving along the seashore is different from open water survival and is not covered by this book; this is when you will be glad you packed something like *The Sea Survival Manual* in your grab bag, or have something similar on your phone or tablet. Food and water are usually more abundant ashore, and shelter easier to locate and construct. With the immediate problems of survival solved, rescue again becomes the priority. It is important to make use of any and all possible methods of attracting attention, including two methods that were not available in your liferaft. They are signal fires and ground to air signalling.

Signal fires

Establish signal fires as soon as possible. Ideally, build three fires in a triangle at equal distances apart and kept them dry and maintained. Do not light the fires until you see an aircraft or vessel, unless fuel is abundant.

Create smoke to contrast with your background:

- For light smoke against dark earth or forest – use green leaves, damp grass, seaweed etc.
- For dark smoke against snow or desert sand – use rubber, such as bits of liferaft etc.

Ground-to-air signalling

Construct signs as large and noticeable as possible, ideally 10m (30ft) for each letter, and each line 2m (6ft) wide. Make the letters in as clear an area as possible, using a colour that contrasts with the ground. Use one of the following:

- **V** – I require assistance.
- **X** – I require medical assistance.

Leaving the beaching area

Once the signalling fires and signs are organised and all the distress alerting equipment from aboard the liferaft has been made ready, you can consider the future. Explore the area for any clear signs of inhabitation or an obvious direction where help might be located. If there is nothing to indicate anyone nearby then it may be better to stay where you landed, especially if food and water are available. If you do decide that all or one of you should go for help, where to go will be determined by any information you have gathered or knowledge of the area. If all else fails, follow the coast or a waterway.

▶ Appendix 1

VOYAGE DETAILS PLAN

Details of Vessel

Name of vessel:

Builder:	Model:	LOA:

Registered owner:

Port of registry:	Official no:

Description of Vessel

Type: **Motor / Sail**	Rig: **Schooner / Ketch / Sloop**

Colour of sails:	Colour of topsides:
Colour of hull above waterline:	Colour of hull below waterline:

Where name displayed:

Any special identifying features:

Engine Type:	No. of engines:
HP:	Fuel capacity:
Dinghy make and model:	Dinghy colour:

Skipper of Vessel

Name:	DOB:

Address:

Mobile:	Nautical qualifications:
PLB make & model:	No:

Any additional information:

Life-saving Equipment

Lifejacket type:	No:	Colour:
Lifejacket type:	No:	Colour:
Liferaft make and model:		Liferaft colour:
Liferaft emergency pack:		Grab bag contents list attached: **YES / NO**
Flares carried (excluding inside liferaft)	orange smoke no:	red handheld no:
red parachute no:	white parachute no:	LED:
1st EPIRB make:	model:	serial no:
2nd EPIRB make:	model:	serial no:
SART: **YES / NO**	AIS: **YES / NO**	

Radio and Navigation Equipment

Fixed VHF make & model:	DSC: **YES / NO**
Radio callsign:	MMSI no.
1st Portable VHF make & model:	DSC: **YES / NO**
2nd Portable VHF make & model:	DSC: **YES / NO**
Satellite system make & model:	Phone no:
MF/HF: **YES / NO**	Radar: **YES / NO**	Echo sounder: **YES / NO**

VOYAGE DETAILS PLAN (continued)

Planned Trip

Date of departure:	Time:
Departure from:	
Way stop 1:	ETA:
Way stop 2:	ETA:
Final destination:	ETA:
Possible alternative ports:	
Other information:	

Crew/Passengers Aboard

Number of persons aboard:

Name:	DOB:
Mobile:	Health issue:
PLB make & model:	Registered to:
Emergency contact:	Tel no:
Name:	DOB:
Mobile:	Health issue:
PLB make & model:	Registered to:
Emergency contact:	Tel no:
Name:	DOB:
Mobile:	Health issue:
PLB make & model:	Registered to:
Emergency contact:	Tel no:
Name:	DOB:
Mobile:	Health issue:
PLB make & model:	Registered to:
Emergency contact:	Tel no:
Name:	DOB:
Mobile:	Health issue:
PLB make & model:	Registered to:
Emergency contact:	Tel no:

Additional Information:

What to do if vessel is overdue

If no contact made by:

Call the Coastguard or Local Authority on:

If you need to contact us while we are underway:

Notes: *This passage plan has been left with you and only with you, as I know you can be relied upon to contact the number(s) above if necessary. If for any reason our departure is delayed, I promise to phone you immediately so our expected arrival date can be changed. I also promise to phone you as soon as possible should there be any other change of plan, and immediately upon our arrival at each stop.*

▶ *Appendix 2*

MAYDAY VHF PROCEDURE

**Motor/Yacht Serenity
November Hotel Golf Whisky 8
MMSI 366924365**

IF THE VESSEL OR A PERSON IS IN GRAVE AND IMMINENT DANGER AND IMMEDIATE ASSISTANCE IS REQUIRED:

VHF/DSC Radio

- Check VHF is on. (If not, depress green button).
- Remove handset from wall unit.
- Lift plastic lid, on wall unit, covering orange button.
- **PRESS AND HOLD ORANGE 'DISTRESS' BUTTON FOR 5 SECONDS.**
- Wait and listen.
  On receipt of an acknowledgement, or after 15 seconds:
- Press red 'CH 16' button.
- If 'LOW' is displayed on screen, press 'HI/LO' button.
- **PRESS TRANSMIT BUTTON**, and say slowly and clearly:
  MAYDAY, MAYDAY, MAYDAY
  This is Serenity, Serenity, Serenity.
  Mayday Serenity, November Hotel Golf Whisky Eight. MMSI 366924365
- **My position is ….** (latitude and longitude using GPS).
- **IF YOU DON'T KNOW, DON'T GUESS!**
- **I am ….** (sinking, on fire etc.)
- **I require immediate assistance**
- **I have …** (number of persons on board, any other information – drifting, flares fired etc.)
- **Over**

- **RELEASE THE TRANSMIT BUTTON** and listen for an acknowledgement.
- **KEEP LISTENING ON CH 16 FOR INSTRUCTIONS**

If an acknowledgement is not received, then repeat the distress call process from the beginning. Consider repeating the call on a different channel.

This is an example of a Mayday VHF procedure appertaining to a particular radio. Everything printed in tinted letters should be altered to reflect the equipment and details for your yacht. Any extra instruction, relevant to your particular equipment, should be included to enable a novice to make a successful Mayday call.

▶ *Appendix 3*
SOURCES OF SUPPLIES AND INFORMATION

GOVERNMENT, ORGANISATIONS ETC

Australian Maritime Safety Authority (AMSA)
Australian equivalent of MCA in the UK.
To register 406 MHz EPIRB: AusSAR,
Australian Maritime Safety Authority,
GPO Box 2181, Canberra ACT 2601,
Australia
Tel: +61 (0)2 6279 5766
www.amsa.gov.au

Canada Marine Transportation
Oversees marine safety in Canada for both recreational and commercial vessel safety.
www.tc.canada.ca/en/
marine-transportation/marine-safety

COSPAS-SARSAT
Download USA406 MHz EPIRB registration form and learn lots more about the system.
NOAA SARSAT Beacon Registration
Database
Tel: (toll free) +1 888 212 7283
www.cospas-sarsat.org and www.sarsat.
noaa.gov

Cruising Association
A non-commercial UK organisation representing the interests of cruising sailors worldwide. It makes available up-to-date cruising information and promotes cruising interests.
CA House, 1 Northey Street, Limehouse
Basin, London, E14 8BT, UK
Tel: +44 (0)207 537 2828
www.theca.org.uk

International Maritime Organization (IMO)
United Nations specialised agency responsible for improving marine safety and preventing pollution from ships.
4 Albert Embankment, London,
SE1 7SR, UK
Tel: +44 (0)20 7735 7611
www.imo.org

Inmarsat
Intergovernmental, global, mobile satellite communications operator, allowing voice, data, text and distress communication at sea.
Inmarsat Ltd, 99 City Road, London,
EC1Y 1AX, UK
Tel: +44 (0)207 728 1000
www.inmarsat.com

The Maritime and Coastguard Agency (MCA)
Government agency and controlling body authority for British registered ships, responsible for marine safety, pollution prevention and responding to maritime emergency. Free download of Ship Captain's Medical Guide and most M Notices. (MSN 1726 has a very useful list of drugs and how to use them etc.)
Spring Place, 105 Commercial Road,
Southampton, SO15 1EG, UK
Tel: +44 (0)2380 329100
To register a UK 406 MHz EPIRB: The
EPIRB Registry, MCA Southern Region
(Falmouth), Pendennis Point, Castle
Drive, Falmouth, Cornwall, TR11 4WZ, UK
www.mcagency.org.uk

National Oceanic and Atmospheric Administration (NOAA)
Excellent internet site for USA marine weather, hurricane warnings etc with links to other parts of the organisation.
www.noaa.gov (main site)
www.nws.noaa.gov (National Weather Service home page)

Oyster Rallies
Organiser of round the world rallies for owners of Oyster Yachts.
The Outlook, Fox's Marina, Ipswich, Suffolk, IP2 8NJ, UK
Tel: +44 (0)1473 851436
www.oysteryachts.com/
oyster-world-rally

Royal National Lifeboat Institution (RNLI)
A British organisation to preserve life and promote safety at sea, using lifeboats manned by volunteers and funded by voluntary contributions.
West Quay Road, Poole, Dorset, BH15 1HZ, UK
Tel: +44 (0) 1202 663234
www.rnli.org.uk

Royal Yachting Association (RYA)
A UK organisation, a governing body representing the interests of everyone who goes on the water for pleasure. They run extensive training schemes, including an excellent sea survival course.
RYA House, Ensign Way, Hamble, Southampton, SO31 4YA, UK
Tel: +44 (0)23 80 604100
www.rya.org.uk

The Stationery Office
Publishers of all Acts and Statutory Instruments in force in the UK and applicable to British registered vessels, including pleasure vessels. Recent legislation is available via the website.

Publications Centre, PO Box 29, Norwich, NR3 1GN, UK
Tel: +44 (0)333 202 5070
www.hmso.gov.uk/stat.htm
www.tso.co.uk

The United Kingdom Hydrographic Office (UKHO)
Admiralty Way, Taunton, Somerset, TA1 2DN, UK
Tel: +44 (0)1823 484444
www.admiralty.co.uk

United States Coast Guard (USCG)
A huge, but somewhat confusing site, lots of interesting and useful information on everything to do with the sea and safety.
www.uscg.mil

Viking Maritime Marine Safety Academy
Courses in Basic Safety Training, Sea Survival, Personal Survival Techniques.
Menzies Road, Whitfield, Dover, Kent, CT16 2FG, UK
Tel: +44 (0)300 303 8393
www.maritimeskillsacademy.com

World Cruising
A UK-based sailing organisation that organises several offshore cruising events, including the Atlantic Rally for Cruisers (ARC).
120 High Street, Cowes, Isle of Wight, PO31 7AX, UK
Tel. +44 (0)1983 296060
www.worldcruising.com

World Sailing
World governing body for the sport of sailing, officially recognised by the International Olympic Committee (IOC).
Office 401, 4th Floor, 3 Shortlands Drive, London, W6 8DA, UK
www.sailing.org

DISTRESS EQUIPMENT MANUFACTURERS AND SUPPLIERS

ACR and Artex
Epirbs, ELTs, PLBs, VHF Radios, SARTs, survivor location lights.
Head Office: 5757 Ravenswood Road, Ft. Lauderdale, Florida, 33312, USA
Tel: +1 954 981 3333
www.acrartex.com

ICS Electronics Ltd
Marine safety products including GMDSS systems, Navtex.
Unit V, Rudford Industrial Estate, Ford, Arundel, West Sussex, BN18 0BD, UK
Tel: +44 (0)1903 731101
www.icselectronics.co.uk

Katadyn Products Inc
Portable hand-operated emergency watermakers.
Pfäffikerstrasse 37, 8310, Kemptthal, Switzerland
Tel: +41 44 839 21 11
http://katadyngroup.com

Pains-Wessex
Emergency electronics (EPIRB, VHF, SART), pyrotechnics and survivor location lights.
Wescom Group, Draycott, Derby, DE72 3QJ, UK
Tel: +44 (0)1332 871100
www.painswessex.com

Sartech Engineering Ltd
Marine safety sales and servicing, including Kanard and McMurdo EPIRBs and SARTs.
13 Trowers Way, Holmethorpe Industrial Estate, Redhill, RH1 2LH, UK
Tel: +44 (0)1737 372670
www.sartech.co.uk

LIFERAFT MANUFACTURERS AND DISTRIBUTORS

Ocean Safety
Distributors and service agents of leisure and commercial liferafts.
Branches in Southampton, Plymouth, Greenock and Aberdeen.
Tel: +44 (0)23 8072 0800
www.oceansafety.com

Portland Pudgy
A rugged, unsinkable dinghy you can row, motor, sail and even use as a lifeboat.
125 John Roberts Road, Suite 23 South Portland, Maine, 04106, USA
Tel: +1 207 761 2428
www.portlandpudgy.com

Survitec Zodiac
www.surviteczodiac.com

Switlik Parachute Company
1325 East State Street, Trenton, New Jersey, 08609, USA
Tel: +1 609 587 3300
www.switlik.com

Viking
Head Office: Saedding Ringvej 13, 6710 Esbjerg V, Denmark
Tel: +45 76 11 81 00
www.viking-life.com

Winslow Liferaft Company
11700 SW Winslow Drive, Lake Suzy, Florida, 34269, USA
Tel: 1 800 838 3012 or: +1 941 613 6666
www.winslowliferaft.com

OTHER MANUFACTURERS AND SUPPLIERS

BCB Limited
Medical supplier, both drugs and equipment.
Howell House, Lamby Industrial Park, Wentloog Ave, CF3 2EX, UK
Tel: + 44 (0)29 2043 3700
www.bcbin.com

Cosmo Synthetic Paper
Replacement for paper in applications where durability and longevity are desired.
www.cosmosyntheticpaper.com

J L Darling Corp
All-weather writing paper and pens, including Dura Waterproof Rite paper for use in photocopiers and laser printers.
2614 Pacific Highway East, Tacoma, Washington, 98424, USA
Tel: +1 253 922 5000
www.riteintherain.com

WeatherWriter
All-weather writing paper and pens including waterproof paper for use in photocopiers and laser printers.
Pettaugh, Stowmarket, Suffolk, IP14 6AX, UK
Tel: +44 (0)1473 890285
www.weatherwriter.co.uk

SURVIVAL SITES ON THE INTERNET

Equipped to Survive
Site with information on outdoor gear, survival equipment and survival techniques.
www.equipped.org

Air Cavalry
Site mainly about helicopters, and it includes a good book on survival.
www.aircav.com/survival/asurtoc.html

Maritime Skills Academy (MSA)
Courses in Basic Safety Training, Sea Survival, Personal Survival Techniques.
www.maritimeskillsacademy.com

US Search and Rescue Task Force
A private volunteer organisation on the east coast of the USA. The site contains excellent search and rescue and disaster related information.
www.ussartf.org

▶ *Index*

▶ *Photo Credits*

Viking Maritime Group: 1, 2, 3, 4, 21, 22, 26, 78

ACR Electronics Inc.: 5, 6, 10, 11, 12, 28, 32 (bottom), 34 (top), 55, 57, 84, 85, 96, 98

Inmarsat: 7, 8 (top)

Ocean Safety Ltd: 8 (bottom), 9, 15, 17, 18 (bottom), 19, 20, 24, 31, 33, 35, 36, 37, 38, 39, 41, 42, 43, 45 (bottom), 46, 49, 52, 69, 71, 72, 75, 77, 82, 89, 91, 92, 100, 118, 119

Portland Pudgy, Inc.: 18 (top)

Echomax: 32 (top), 45 (top)

Retevis: 34 (bottom)

Adobe Stock: 47, 51, 58, 79, 107, 115, 120

Frances & Michael Howorth: 67, 99, 109

Gun fired at
intervals of
about a minute

Continuous
sounding of fog-
signalling equipment

Red stars from
a rocket or shell

SOS:
Flashlight – night
Signal mirror – day

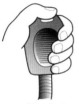

'Mayday'
spoken over the
VHF or SSB

Flags: N & C flown
from the signal halyard

Any square flag
and the anchor
ball, for example

Flames on
the yacht

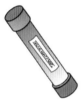

Red parachute
flare (or hand flare)

Orange-coloured
smoke signal,
handheld or floating

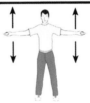

Slowly raise
and lower
outstretched arms

Radiotelephone
alarm signal
on 2182kHz

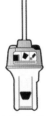

Activate the
406MHz or
Inmarsat E EPIRB

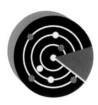

Activate the
radar transponder
(SART)

Orange canvas with
black square
and circle

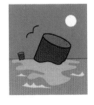

Dye marker of
any colour